I0450359

Pedro Eloy

MY HEALTH, MY LIFE

Roadmap to a Healthy Lifestyle

All rights reserved

Copyright © 2012
Pedro Eloy

All rights reserved. No part of this book may be
reproduced in any form, except for the inclusion of a
brief quotation in a review, without the permission in
writing of the author.

To purchase further copies of *My Health My Life*,
visit Amazon (Amazon.com), Barnes & Noble
(www.barnesandnoble.com) or Alibris
(www.alibris.com) and type in the title of the book
or the Author's name on the website search box.

To view all publications or to contact the author, visit:
www.TheStarBody.com

ISBN-13: 978-1463572914
ISBN-10: 1463572913

My Health, My Life is dedicated to my mother Maria Madalena and to my sister Madalena. No matter the distance, you are and will always be in my heart.

Table of Contents

Part IV - Nutrition: healthier choices

Part V - Final notes: the starting point

Part VI - Useful resources

FOREWORD

BY SADE ADELEKAN
CEO & MANAGING EDITOR
HYDROGEN MAGAZINE, LOS ANGELES, USA

There is a saying, "The proof is in the pudding." With author, entrepreneur and fitness authority Pedro Eloy, this could not be truer. A few years back, I managed a fashion magazine and was looking for someone who could dispense health and fitness advice to my readers in a way that struck the right balance between providing substantive information and direction, and being palatable to a savvy audience whose attention is not easy to capture. Enter Pedro Eloy, the only man that came to mind because of the breadth and depth of his knowledge on the subject, and a man whom I continue to call upon to dispense his knowledge of health and fitness to my HYDROGEN Magazine readers.

I was delighted when Pedro began working on *My Health, My Life*, because this fascinating guide to living a healthy life is told through the eyes and experiences of a man who lives the principles espoused in this page turner, staying active and maintaining a healthy lifestyle while enjoying it every step of the way.

Why, you might ask, is Eloy the right source to go to for knowledge and enlightenment of healthy living? For that, you need to know his background.

Pedro Eloy is sought after by multi-national corporations for his business acumen and expertise in New Media. Add to that a lifelong passion for keeping fit and staying healthy, which led him to start London-based *The Star Body*, an integrative mind-body wellness approach with a track record of helping to transform the bodies and life-outlook of his clients. Highly respected in the H&F industry, Pedro's bold approach taps into the latest trends in proven medical research which he streamlines into an easily adaptable fitness and health regimen anyone can adopt.

My Health, My Life lays out in a compulsively readable fashion, a roadmap to a healthy and enjoyable life. The genius here is not only in the well-researched and in-depth analysis of what will get you on the right road to optimal health and longevity, but Eloy does it with clarity and a sincerity that is evident.

I read *My Health, My Life* sitting on my pool deck on a typically beautiful Los Angeles day...not a bad way to go about it! A couple of chapters particularly resonated with me. My struggle, as with many women I know, is a feeling of being overwhelmed and confused about which diet is the right one and how much or how little exercise I need.

The 'aha' moment for me was learning to change my nutritional paradigms about what I like and dislike. My mind opened up and I started playing a new record in my head, so to speak. Instead of saying to myself, "That bag of chips is the only thing that will satisfy me right now because it tastes so damn good," I learned to look at healthy alternatives. I learned to experiment and derive pleasure from food while making good choices for myself.

I got up from my pool deck that Saturday afternoon saying to myself, "Okay, I can do this!" And I think that is the same feeling others will walk away with after delving into *My Health, My Life,* and I have Pedro Eloy to thank for that.

PREFACE

BY PEDRO ELOY
TO YOUR HEALTH AND WELLNESS

TO YOUR HEALTH AND WELLNESS

"If we could give every individual the right amount
of nourishment and exercise, not too little and not too
much, we would find our way to health"
Hippocrates

Your health is your most valuable investment. You can
live healthy productive years simply by applying a
handful of principles mentioned in this book; in fact,
according to experts, one hundred-plus years of activity
and vitality should be the attainable goal for mankind.
All other mammals live five times the number of years
it takes their skeleton to reach maturity - man reaches
his skeletal maturity at the age of twenty six - this
indicates one hundred years of productive life as a
reasonable goal for all of us.

We have all heard countless times about "eating 5 a
day" and the importance of doing exercise on a regular
basis to look good, young, healthy and to achieve that
long-desired body shape. The facts show that the
number of obesity and weight-gain related illnesses has

been skyrocketing, especially in the so-called modern societies, where the information about how to keep healthy is splattered all over national media.

Plastic surgery has seeped into pop culture, with the growing number of reality TV shows, tabloid breaking news and rumors of celebrities getting different types of cosmetic procedures. The growth in this trend is not limited to the US and UK; people all over the world are doing it to alter specific features and achieve that perfect look and body shape.

The rising supply and demand in the cosmetic surgery industry is undeniable and therefore perpetuating the trend in urban landscapes. People are searching for both the magic procedures promising immediate results at affordable prices. However, the cost of such procedures becomes, most often than not, larger than anticipated, with severe impact on both body and mental health.

The American Society of Plastic Surgeons reported in 2010 the numbers of weight loss related procedures: 203,106 for Liposuction and 116,352 for Abdominoplasty. Still according to this source, 13.1 million cosmetic procedures, 1.6 million cosmetic surgical procedures and 11.6 million cosmetic minimally-invasive procedures took place in the USA in the same year.

Whilst plastic surgery may be advised for specific aesthetic cases, customized health and fitness programmes can produce outstanding results in the areas of weight-loss and overall body-toning, providing real and consistent results that are sustainable in the long run. The bottom line is that you can lose a considerable amount of weight together with a significant reduction in cellulite by learning how to progressively integrate supporting disciplines - such as nutrition and exercise - into your lifestyle.

Statistical data on the topic of health and wellness also show the ongoing rise of what was once a minor psychological ailment, becoming one of the main reasons for visiting the family doctor: stress. From an evolutionary perspective, stress is related to our fight/flight mechanism; our brain is constantly searching for potential danger in the surroundings, and is ready to mobilize resources and to prompt us for immediate action. The stress response is biphasic, that is, the system meets short-term stress by increasing certain responses, including immunological functions. Sustained stress, unresolved traumas and failure to adapt can seriously impair cognitive functions, down-regulate immune responses and, eventually, create cellular and metabolic damage.

Following many years of natural evolution, the brain has registered the dangers of confronting with deadly predators and other day-to-day threats. In modern societies, one does not have to go hunting with and for ferocious animals that can take one's life in a split of a second. Our fight-and-flight response is still ingrain in our brain and helps to deploy immediate responses to perceived threats, both external - arising from the "real world"- and internal - as a consequence of our thought process that may perceive an emotional alert as a real and urgent threat. Scientific papers on this subject have concluded that this "emergency-mechanism" does not distinguish between modern-world emotional stress and real life-or-death stressful events. In short, the process designed to save our lives in moments of real danger can also cause, especially in emotionally inducted danger occasions, a corrosive and damaging outcome to both our body and mind.

A healthy mindset is as important as a healthy body, or, in other words, feeling good and looking good go hand in hand and cannot exist one without the other. As the body needs to be kept fit and exercised, so does the mind, and action must also be taken to nurture and care for our mental self.

I believe you will find much to learn from this book; put it all into practice and you can look forward to an enjoyable and healthier life – at any age.

"And in the end it's not the years in your life that count; It's the life in your years" - Abraham Lincoln.

Entrepreneur and fitness aficionado, Pedro Eloy is a specialist in new media & online business, working with top management in multinational organizations.

As a personal passion, Pedro Eloy has been researching, teaching and sharing about health and fitness for many years. A true fitness aficionado, Pedro Eloy possesses a solid reputation in the H&F industry being recognized for his innovative and straightforward approach based on the latest trends in medical research. Pedro is the Founder of London-based The Star Body, an integrative concept addressing mind and body as a whole, with a proven track record of delivering fitness excellence. As an author, Pedro Eloy has been a regular contributor to UK and US-based magazines.

Pedro Eloy holds a Diploma in Diet and Nutrition, a CIEH award in Food Safety & Catering and is a Healthy Food Chef specializing in Transitional Cuisine. He is a MP in Neuro-Linguistic Programming and is certified in Clinical & Sports Hypnotherapy. He is a member of the

International Medical and Dental Hypnotherapy Association and the British Longevity Society.

Pedro Eloy works in an international setting. He has lived and worked in Portugal, Canada, USA, UK and Hong Kong.

PART I

STATISTICS AND FACTS

AN EVOLUTIONARY PERSPECTIVE

AN EVOLUTIONARY PERSPECTIVE

Human life span has been a topic of investigation for many years. Three centuries ago, French scientist George-Louis Leclerc de Buffon determined, in his *Histoire Naturelle de l'Homme* that the natural life span of a man was 100-plus years; according to Buffon, all other mammals live to five times the number of years it takes their skeleton to mature - a dog's skeleton matures at three; his normal life is fifteen to sixteen years. A man's skeleton matures at twenty-five/twenty-eight years of age - so 125 years or better are Buffon's estimate of the number of years a man should aspire to live.

Active lives at 100-plus

A growing number of people are living to these ages with vigor and virility today in many parts of the world. Many of us know the story of the Hunza in the Himalayas - these people are living active lives at 120 and more. In Rajshapur, India, many of its citizens also live to advanced years (100-plus) in excellent health. In the last days of Gandhi's life, incidentally, during the riots which eventually saw his assassination, the Mahatma said a most interesting thing. He stated with some prescience of his fate, "I don't think that I shall live to be 125." This comment seems strange to the Western mind, which cannot accept such longevity as a natural goal. But it was in perfect keeping with the Indian experience, since many of them do live to such a great age.

Such basic principles of good health that are being implemented by people all around the world have already tripled our average life spans, as the following shows:

- The estimated average length of life in the early Iron and Bronze Age was about 18 years, according to studies of skeletal remains.

- In Ancient Rome, that average lifespan was about 22 years, in agreement with the indications provided from certain burial inscriptions.

- From the Middle Ages until the time of the American Revolution, little changes occurred in the average lifespan in the Western world although, in many regions, a slight increase to 33 years was the new standard.

Poor sanitation together with little knowledge of preventive medicine were responsible for keeping the average lifespan between 30 to 35 years over the centuries, until the dawn of the industrial age. By the middle of the eighteenth century, lifespan rose to about 40 years and, one-half century later, this average increased again to 49 years in the United States. During the next half-century, the US lifespan rose by nearly 20 years, to reach a level of 68.6 years in 1952.

According to the data from the US National Center for Health Statistics, the average life expectancy for an American born in 2005 increased to 77.6 years, and in 2009, it was raised to 78.2 years representing a further 0.2 years in contrast to data from 2008. This increase in life expectancy has a direct correlation to modern medicine and the advances in public health.

Statistical data

In the last century, we have seen an extraordinary reduction in mortality statistics, for which the control of infections is considered to be the one of the main causes. Contrasts are evident for the situations in the United States in 1900, 1954, 2003 and 2009. At the earlier date, five infectious conditions were heading the list: pneumonia and influenza, with a death rate of 202 per 100,000, tuberculosis with a rate of 194 per 100,000, and diarrhea & enteritis with 143 per 100,000. Diphtheria ranked among the first 10 with a rate of 40 per 100,000.

These few infectious conditions alone accounted for

one-third of all deaths in the United States in the beginning of the 20th century. Fifty years later, death rates from pneumonia and influenza had been reduced to about one-eighth of the 1900's statistics and these two death-related illnesses ranked only sixth amongst the main death causes. By this time, Tuberculosis no longer ranked as a top ten death-related illness and diarrhea, enteritis & diphtheria were now at the bottom of such list.

In 2003, according to the US National Vital Statistic System, the top causes of death were heart-related diseases (28%); cancer (22.7%); cerebrovascular diseases (6.5%); and respiratory diseases (5.2%). Six years later, in 2009, the latest published data show the two main causes of death were still heart-related disease (24.57%) and malignant neoplasms (23.34%), followed by chronic lower respiratory diseases (5.63%) and cerebrovascular diseases (5.28%). Furthermore, from 2008 to 2009, the preliminary adjusted rate for the leading causes of death showed that heart-related diseases decreased by 3.7% and malignant neoplasms by 1.1%.

All these figures show there has been a significant reduction of the common death causes from the 1900's throughout 1950's. In fact, cardiovascular diseases and cancer reached the forefront in the middle of the 20th century and, in 2009, heart diseases and cancer –related illnesses were responsible for 48% of all deaths in the

United States, with influenza and pneumonia ranking eight amongst this list. In conclusion, in the last one-hundred years, there has been an important shift from the so-called and early life-related diseases to the mid-life and older age illnesses.

Following the post-industrial revolution era, the two leading causes for mortality of middle aged individuals were heart-related diseases and cancer, the latter accounting for about 20% of the deaths in the U. S. This figure could be reduced to less than half its present toll if periodic cancer detection examinations had been a national habit, rather than the exceptional effort of a few, as they are now. Periodic health examinations will also help to trace many other diseases which if detected in early stages can drastically increase the success and recovery rates.

The actual tendency shows that the more successful - economically and professionally - a person becomes, the more inactive his or her life is and, consequently, the greater chance he or she has of dying young. The facts show that the more sedentary the occupation, the more dangerous it is: three and one-half times more deaths from hardening of the arteries occur amongst professional businessmen and women when compared to unskilled laborers. Recent statistical data shows that the so-called civilized and sedentary way of living is causing people to die early and and rendering many others unable to work or to have a fully active personal life at early ages. To corroborate this statement, available data show that from the age of 55, about ten per cent of any civilized country's work force is on disability pensions. Many of these early forced retirements are the consequence of strokes, heart attacks, hardening of arteries and flabby muscles. Since physical inactivity is probably the main cause of this invalidism and death, planned exercise programs are one of the key answers and can easily be incorporated into every daily routine and made to fit every lifestyle.

One of the most famous exercise programs conceptualized by Beckmann in the Bavarian mountains (1953) was the "Ohlstadter Kur". This has been a model for similar exercise programs in other parts of Germany, Austria, Greece, Holland, Norway, the former Yugoslavia and Israel.

One other interesting "unofficial exercise program" was implemented in many Swedish companies, where the "coffee break" is replaced by exercise breaks for ten to twenty minutes. Within the office or factory, each group does planned physical activity under the leadership of their supervisor, a person who has been especially trained to conduct this program.

Many countries are now offering four to six-week residential rehabilitation programmes to address the importance of exercise in overall health. Between 1957 and 1959, 86.3% participants in one of these reconditioning centers remained free of illness although the same individuals had been repeatedly ill before that period.

Important work in the United States was done in the past by W. V. Cumler of the Central Branch of the Cleveland YMCA. The following summarizes the results on reducing diastolic blood pressure by means of a model program of calisthenics and running activities. The following conclusions depict the study of four men and the observed results: how an average total of 58 years were added to their life expectancy within a few short months of the illustrated programme:

Subject A

Blood pressure too high and too rapid a pulse. This man's ailments might not seem great on the surface; yet his blood pressure showed he had only one-half the normal life expectancy for his age. In two months of an exercise program his blood pressure decreased to normal values and his life expectancy increased to about thirteen years more.

Subject B

A younger man with significantly high blood pressure had less than a third of normal life expectancy. At the end of his fourth month of exercise he had a more efficient pulse and much better chances for long life -

about eighteen years more.

Subject C

On this man's chart, the blood pressure readings represented the lowest he was able to attain by using certain high-blood-pressure medicines. His physician reminded him of the importance of keeping his nurse informed of his general health as soon as he started the fitness program in order to ensure that his medications remained at a proper level. During the second month of activity, he felt so good he decided to stop taking the medication. In spite of this non-recommended act, his test at the end of the third month showed a normal blood pressure with a truly tremendous increase in life expectancy amounting to twenty extra years.

Subject D

This individual exhibited the most dramatic result variation from the first test to the second. Pulse and both phases of blood pressure had gone from the too-frequently-seen findings of neglected middle age to those of an Olympic athlete. Life expectancy had doubled.

All life expectancies shown above are valid statistical assumptions based on the best prevailing medical information at the time the experiments were performed, in early 1960s.

If there was a single magic pill or "shot" that would immediately assure a long, vigorous life, people would be cueing to purchase it, no matter its cost. At the turn of the nineteenth century, when advertising was in its infancy, in a time where less sophistication and education were common, this promise of "long life in a bottle" was offered by hundreds of salesmen. In those days, although the product wouldn't work, the promise did. People would rush out and buy snake root, swamp grass, liver bile, or any other nauseating mixture the so-called medicine man had compounded. Today everyone "knows better". The world laughs at the promise of a long, healthy, vigorous life; feeble excuses which only hide our own inner knowledge that we are shortening our lives, deliberately and inevitably. Women do outlive men in the United States, and in much of the Western world. But men outlive women in Finland and in New Zealand. These statistics are only the current, twentieth-century figures on mortality.

After careful reading of different medical opinions, the conclusion is that there is no such thing as a biological superiority of females over males. Whatever hereditary differences there are between men and women, these do not lengthen or shorten life. It is what one does with one's body, and not so much the kind of body one is given, that counts in the long run. There is also the common fear of "overdoing" a fitness program, or of "straining some body part". This can be dispelled with the following facts:

- No one has ever been able to prove the occurrence of a heart attack in an athlete. Athletes out of condition are in the same boat with the rest of us, of course.

- In Finland it has been shown, many times, that those who ski live several years longer than those who do not.

- Physical training not only makes us feel better but it is also *the only way* the body chemistry can be kept in good condition.

One of the reasons people really feel tired in the evening is due to spending the whole day monotonously sitting. We rush home to lie down before bedtime. Too often our motto seems to be: don't stand if you can sit; don't sit if you can lie down. Every day that one increases one's fitness one will gain mental tranquility and physical vigor.

PART II

INNER HEALTH

THE "MAESTRO" INSIDE THE MACHINE
IMPACT OF REAL AND PERCEIVED STRESS
SLEEP & RECOVERY
DREAMLAND *VERSUS* REALITY

THE "MAESTRO" INSIDE THE MACHINE

Dreams of immortal beings or even the many writings on vampire figures that live *ad-eternum* are featured vastly on fictional literature. Without aiming to delve into any religion branch or bringing up atheist theories, the facts show that each human being remains on this earth for a certain number of years. Whilst living, many have asked the question of who is the maestro inside the machine, the control centre that ensures that our hearts beat a certain number of times per day, our blood circulates internally and that the food we eat nourishes our inner organs. The complexity of our internal system has only been partially framed by the medical institution which can provide "body fixtures" only to a certain extent. When entering the field of the mind, the so-called black-box of the human being, assumptions become susceptible to interpretations.

One of the most prominent figures in psychiatry, Sigmund Freud, versed vastly on the three components of what he called the psyche's structural model: the *id* the *ego* and the *super-ego*. According to Freud's model the *id* was the set of uncoordinated instinctual trends; the *ego*, the organized, realistic part; and the *super-ego* playing the critical and moralizing role. The *id* refers to the unorganized part of the personality structure which contains the basic drives - it acts according to the "pleasure principle", seeking to avoid pain or displeasure aroused by increases in instinctual tension. Being the unconscious by definition, *"It is the dark, inaccessible part of our personality, what little we know of it we have learned from our study of the dream-work and of the construction of neurotic symptoms, and most of that is of a negative character and can be described only as a contrast to the ego. We approach the id with analogies: we call it a chaos, a cauldron full of seething excitations... It is filled with energy reaching it from the instincts, but it has no organization, produces no collective will, but only a striving to bring about the satisfaction of the instinctual needs subject to the observance of the pleasure principle."*

Centuries before Freud unveiled his paradigmatic conclusions to this concept, an ancient civilization – the Egyptians - used to gather entire communities in one room where the main holy entity would conduct long sessions of mass trance as a way to address body and mind ailments.

Throughout history, many theoreticians have versed on the subjects of the mind and the inner entity that keeps each of us alive – for the purpose of this chapter and without offending any scientific/non-scientific entity, we will use the term *unconscious* to address the inner self.

The question that immediately arises is whether there is in fact an inner self that somehow manages all internal processes together with our daily energy levels and health state. The answer is that no one knows! The inner self, the maestro inside the machine has not yet been quantifiable or presented in an auditorium for detailed analysis. Just like a black box analysis type much has been done, research wise, to try to understand its own working mechanism. Unlike ordinary machinery, the brain-core that controls all the inner functions did not come with an instruction manual.

The keys to the unconscient mind

The unconscious mind has been the focus of several scientific and non-scientific studies to provide a better understanding of its *modus operandum* mechanism. Described as a *black box* per nature, its conclusions are based on the outputs produced during experiments done within this field, some of which are summarized below:

- It stores and organizes temporal and atemporal memories: it also sorts and catalogues all the flavored experiences - our perceptions of reality.

Memories can be re-flavored every time we bring them to our conscient screen, based on new assumptions and what is accept as the "new truth".

- It is the domain of emotions. Neural pathways are constantly being created and re-created to provide interpretations, explanations and re-interpretations of daily experiences.

- It provides access and references to past experiences allowing us to take immediate decisions. The "yellow flag" on this note is that what we may have recorded and archived as a lesson from a past experience may in fact be a distorted version of the reality that is not serving us appropriately, as a reference cue.

- May keep negative memories with negative emotions archived & repressed. It may also release them into the conscient screen when appropriate in an attempt to "let go" – the so-called "release of repressed memories".

- It runs the body in its entirety. It runs the organs, the heart, the lungs and internal mechanisms such as digestion and production of white blood cells. If we had to do all these internal operations consciently, we would probably not have time to do anything else with our lives.

- Its primary goal is to keep the integrity of the body, hence the existence of our own "chatter box" whose mission is to keep us safe and within a so-called "comfort zone".

- Supports the morality and the *status quo* that we were taught have chosen to accept, consciently or unconsciently through repetition by authority figures such as our parents and school teachers.

- It's a servant and likes to follow orders. It is like a child - whatever we give it to play, it will entertain - each entertained thought creates an imprint in our memory banks. This imprint will have an emotional charge (colors, odors, flavors...) that we have associated to it. The more one entertains any thought, the bigger the imprint in our memory banks and the greater the impact it will have in our lives. One actually becomes what one thinks about most of the times; the thoughts given to one's mind to be entertained will greatly contribute to one's present and upcoming reality. The more the mind re-plays a memory, the stronger the assumption and the deeper it will impact.

- It is the gatekeeper of all perceptions. This is probably where the greatest paradox of life comes into play: the contrast between overall reality and the individual perceived facts that each of us repackages to become one's own perception of reality. Upon the confrontation with any piece of information that is detected by our sensory organs, there is the need to explain and to interpret this information packet; an example of this this is when looking at an object that has four legs, a seat and back support - we automatically call it "a chair". What we are actually doing is, upon facing this information packet captured by our eyes, we automatically go into our memory reference index to see if there is any similar object that may have resemblances; we therefore distort and generalize it to provide immediate meaning to what we are experiencing. Due to the amount of information captured at any given second by our sensory organs, there is the need to delete much of it otherwise we would spend our limited 24 hours per day just to interpret, catalogue and make sense of all that surrounds us.

- It is responsible for all the internal energy management.

- It maintains instincts – primarily the survival instincts that have been imprinted many centuries ago, such as the *fight-flight instinct.*

- It is programmed to know and learn always more.

- Uses and responds to symbolism, hence its extensive usage on political and advertising campaigns (ex: the repeated usage of a logo and its colors).

- It takes "everything" personally and will work on the principle of least effort. It also does not process negatives.

The story of the two monks and a woman

This is a very well known Zen story. There are many versions but its origin is not clear...

A senior and a junior monk were traveling somewhere in the high mountains in China. At one point, they met with a river which had a very strong current. As the two monks were preparing to cross this river, they saw a very young and beautiful woman also attempting to cross it. The young woman immediately asked if they could help her to cross this river.

The senior monk carried this woman on his right shoulder and let her down once on the other side. The junior monk was very upset, but said nothing.

Whilst walking, the senior monk noticed that his junior was rather silent and asked "Is there something wrong? You seem very upset." The junior monk replied, "As monks, we are not permitted a woman, so how could you carry that woman on your shoulders?" to which the senior monk replied, "I left the woman a long time ago at the bank, however, you seem to be carrying her still."

The younger monk was bound by ideas and held on to them for hours. In doing so he missed the experiences of the next part of a journey.

There is a tremendous amount of misleading folklore concerning self-care and health. As intelligent people, we want to do what is best, but the folklore interferes. Let's look at some of our most common twenty first century fables in the light of facts.

Stress

Stress is being blown out of proportion. Not only can we tolerate difficulties in our daily living, but in fact we actually need them. The kind of stress that kills occurred far more frequently when our ancestors lived in caves with only a stick to protect them from ferocious creatures. They lived through it and learned how to turn these animals into food, oil, clothes and body ornaments in the process, thus bettering themselves in every way.

On the other side of this equation, severe mental stress cannot only lead to a personality breakdown but also to the path of an Einstein. For the most, it can be the spur that forces us to solve and learn from personal problems with satisfaction and joy rather than being painful hurdles we hope that are solved by someone else.

Many years ago the Greek philosophers observed that there should be "moderation in all things," and moderation is our defense against stress. When too much stress comes our way in one direction, we should look for tasks (or even trains of thoughts) that lead us into another direction. This was what Freud meant when he talked of sublimation: if one task or one situation overwhelms you with tension, walk out on it; go out and take a good walk, swim or play a game of, say, tennis. You need some physical outlet to blow off steam and then come back fresh and unwound. The trouble may still be waiting for you - or it may have gone away during your absence, as it so often surprisingly does.

Stress and the drives of life are inseparable. The way to win the battle with stress is by preparation, onslaught and renewal to attack again; not by retiring to a life in a cocoon of cotton candy and inactivity. Taking up a hobby or a specialized study that is of interest will give us another outlet in which to put our stress to work, rather than being overwhelmed by it.

Dealing with real and perceived stress

From an evolutionary perspective, stress is related to our fight-flight mechanism. Our brain is constantly searching for potential danger in the surroundings and ready to mobilize one's resources or prompt us for immediate action. Following many years of natural evolution, our brain has registered the dangers of confronting with deadly predators and other day-to-day dangers that man has been dealing with and adapting to.

The areas of our brain responsible for prompting us to take immediate action are very quick-tempered. They usually hijack the slow-paced reasoning of our frontal cortex as this swiftness of action may be the difference between life and death. This mechanism, constantly analysing our surroundings and ready to intervene in a split of a second has, as its primary focus, the mission of keeping us in safe boundaries. Whenever the "alarm" is strong enough, our "protective fight-flight brain area" hijacks activity away from rational thought and trusts entirely on an automatic emergency rescue-type response. Have you ever been driving and find yourself suddenly pressing the breaks only to realize you have avoided an accident with another car without even noticing the close presence of it? This is a classic example of the behavioural hijack of our primitive "fight-or-flight" system when it senses immediate danger. Can you imagine what would happen if one was to initially access the situation logically before taking some form of abrupt action? Before we had reached a conclusion and taken any kind of action... it would have probably been too late.

Our emergency-mode is internally activated: the hypothalamus sends an alarm signal to the adrenal glands, generating a multitude of simultaneous responses. These glands will immediately release adrenaline and, as a consequence, the heart rate goes up, blood is sent to the muscles the organs and to the brain which, together with the lungs, is flooded with oxygen. To provide us with quick energy to fuel the needed reaction, glucose is released and fatty acids are mobilized as a quick source of energy. The vessels near the surface of the skin contract and the blood clothing ability is increased in case the "event" may involve bleeding. At the same time, endorphins lock into cell receptors to block the eventual sensation of pain.

Once the fight-or-flight mechanism kicks in, one becomes hyper-alert and ready to respond to the upcoming threat. Time seems to slow down as our brain synapses go into overdrive and our vision alters, ready to detect any dangerous movement in the proximity.

The aftermath

Following a stressful episode, our body will enter the so-called "compensation mode" so that it can go back to a desirable balance. The body has suffered an intense chemical challenge and begins its repair mode. Cortisol, a steroid hormone derived from cholesterol, will start an anti-inflammatory activity and will help to restore the depleted energy sources, together with aiding with the delivery of white blood cells to any injured area. Cortisol also assists with other internal functions to bring the event to the long term memory for future reference - a process also known as stress-enhanced memory.

The stress response is biphasic, that is, the system meets short-term stress by increasing certain responses including immunological functions. Sustained stress, unresolved traumas and failure to adapt can seriously impair cognitive functions, down-regulate immune output and, eventually, create cellular and metabolic damage. In short, the process designed to save our lives in moments of real or emotionally perceived danger, is also a corrosive and damaging to both our body and mind. In modern societies, one does not have to go hunting for ferocious animals that can take our life in a split second; still, our fight-and-flight response acts as a defence system to both real and perceived threats where the latter is a consequence of our thought process that may perceive any emotional alert as a real and urgent threat.

The self-regulating mechanism that seeks to restore

order after stressful events is often referred to as "homeostasis", a word which suggests that the body has a set internal state to which it must return to maintain balance and health. One definition for dynamic health may be our ability to respond to challenges and the speed we regain homeostasis.

Animal studies show that encounters with predators in the wild triggers much the same physiological response as humans experience when facing acute stress - real or emotional. A stressful episode in the animal world is often accompanied by a rush of endorphins, presumably to minimize the pain of being torn apart which sometimes is followed by immobility – the freeze alternative to the fight-or-flight response. Should the prey escape, something interesting occurs: escaping from an ultimate death causes the animal to stay frozen for a while and then being seized by a series of tremors that may mimic the act of running away, followed by a series of uncontrollable muscle spasms. After a few moments, the animal will go back to his normal existence almost as if nothing has happened. As far as we know, these events do not cause the animal any stress-related organ issues, or long-term psychosis and consequent need to end up on a psychiatrist's couch.
Ethnologists now agree that the animal fast recovery from these events is due to their ability to quickly release stress; failure to dissipate this emotional charge

or even carrying it for longer periods may result in mental and body damage, together with potential internal dysfunctions.

The Russian-born Nobel Prize winner Ilya Prigogine concluded that energetic challenges (such as stress) drive the system effectively until it reaches a point of maximum tolerance. This rise of our immune response reaches a point where this system either collapses in growing disorder or dissipates enough energy to safely return to homeostasis. The same way our brain keeps storing life-threatening events - or perceived ones such as strong negative emotions - for future reference, it can also store reinterpretations of the same emotional events by detaching their emotional charge (just like zebras do following a life threatening attack) and link a valuable lesson to that memory. Unresolved incidents stored in our memory banks keep popping into our conscient screen only to be dragged back into the unconscious storage until the day we are able to deal with them and release the associated emotional charge - the so called "let-go process".

Mental fatigue

Mental fatigue responds best to a change of mental scenery. No one has ever demonstrated this better than Sir Isaac Newton. He was completely stumped on a mathematics problem, and decided to go for a walk in his garden. There he saw the fall of an apple and realized the concept of gravity - a momentous discovery made by a mentally-fatigued brain. We don't always need the garden walk to change our mental scenery, but we do need the willingness to change our train of thoughts in order to achieve clarity and mental stability.

Emotional disorders, particularly depressions, are largely responsible for progressively self-destruction. By depression, physicians mean a deep-seated feeling of unworthiness and despair. Such a condition can arise quite suddenly "out of nowhere," and be just as fatal as another depression that has lasted for years. Its recognition is the key to treatment.

In studying people who are ninety and more, the so-called *successful agers*, one common trait stands out: these individuals share a common mental outlook. This mental attitude has been taught in the writings of thoughtful men from China, India, Greece, and other cradles of civilization. These writers have tried to impart certain methods of living life well and to the fullest. If the only result of using these principles was a long life, many people might not want to attempt a change in their thoughts and habits, but the gain from this specific mental outlook is more than a longer life. It is a better, happier and fulfilling daily life.

This is not a philosophy of denial, but of discovery.

Fear of making this discovery has undoubtedly caused greater unhappiness and grief than any positive act ever has. The first step in this is the motto revealed on a column of the ancient Greek temple of Apollo: "Know Thyself". In our daily life, we put a fair amount of time and study into seeking knowledge from others. The salesman wants to know his customers' weaknesses and strengths; the employee who studies the boss in order to improve his chances for promotion; the manager who seeks out ways of improving work through better relationships with his subordinates. We are all busy studying each other and part of this obsession may be an attempt to keep us from discovering and focusing on ourselves.

As twenty first century citizens, we feel that this knowledge is perhaps too ancient and distant to be of much use in the present. Epictetus, Marcus Aurelius, and other philosophers in their many writings point out the benefits of mental-related practices and activities. Even today, the growing fascination with Yoga is certainly due to the fact that this philosophy can assist men and women with their overall self.

The highest mental effort - contemplation - brings forth great rewards. The dictionary gives us a first definition which is needlessly strict: "Meditation on spiritual things." Because of this, many feel that contemplation is a mental act reserved for saints and hermits. There is however a second definition which may be more appropriate: "Contemplation is an act of considering with attention; musing; study." Actually, contemplation occurs when we keep our attention fixed on an object causing the brain, like a machine, to continue searching, and producing a new combination of scenarios and answers through its memory banks, to what is being contemplated. These answers may be called intuition, serendipity or illumination, depending upon the frame of reference.

It's not the content it's the setting.

One of my business partners once came into my practice in Berkley Square, London, with a truly unhappy face. She stepped in and went straight to the balcony. Despite my attempts to get her cheered up she told me that we needed to talk.

My unconscious mind started to think that there could actually be a real and unpleasant problem and begun to prepare my body with internal chemistry, ready to go into an "argumentative mode"…. my body was getting ready for the battle that somehow was heading my way. This escalated into affecting the clarity of my thoughts, retrieving past archived perceived events from my memory banks that could somehow provide any background for what could be coming. I could have thought that nothing was actually wrong and that it all could be just a minor issue, but by having my body gearing up into a fight-flight state, the clarity of my thoughts was truly being affected thus diminishing my chances of calmly resolving any upcoming challenge... The interesting fact was that all this gearing-up was automatically happening without my conscient self having the slightest clue of what this was all about!

In the end, I listened to the so-called major issue and clearly noticed that there was actually no life-threatening situation whatsoever and, for a second, noticed what was happening inside my body – I was actually geared up for war. This status could have in fact been an enabler to a discussion that did not needed to have happened and that did not happen in the end.

It is interesting to analyze, in retrospective, that even the slightest move that may indicate some sort of personal danger can cause both parties to fire their weapons until there is no more ammunition inside the barrels, just like in a action movie where both sides are ready to pull the trigger.....and then someone sneezes....ending up in total massacre!

In such films, after both parties have fired all their bullets, there is a time when the director says "cut" meaning it is time for all the actors to stand up and laugh about the situation! In contrast, this may not be the case in real life. In many circumstances, the amount of psychological bullets that have been fired may not allow the parties involved to go back to a pleasant environment and benefit from a healthy relationship.

To whom does *the gift* belong?

There once lived a great warrior. Though quite old, he was still able to defeat any challenger, both physically and verbally. His reputation extended far and wide and many youngsters gathered to study under him.

One day a well-known infamous young warrior arrived at the village. He was determined to be the first to defeat the great master. Along with his strength, he had an uncanny ability to spot and exploit weaknesses in his so-called opponents. He would wait for his opponent to make the first move, thus revealing a weakness, and then would strike with merciless force and lightning speed.

Much against the advice of his students, the old master accepted the young warrior's challenge. The young warrior began to hurl insults at the old master; he threw dirt and spit in his face; he verbally assaulted him with every curse and insult known to mankind for hours... but the old warrior merely stood there, motionless and calm. Finally, the young warrior exhausted himself. Knowing he was defeated, he left feeling shamed.

Somewhat disappointed that he did not fight the insolent youth, the students gathered around the old master and questioned him. "How could you endure such an indignity?

The old master, after cleaning himself, portrayed a pleasant calm smile and reverted: "If someone comes to give you a gift and you do not receive it, to whom does the gift belong?"

How much sleep do we need for vibrant health? Newspapers seem to confound our ordinary impressions about the necessity of sleep with reports of elderly people who went without sleep for most of their lives. These people are the geniuses - the rare exceptions that can be admired, but should not be imitated. Sleep is a necessity of life, not a luxury: too little sleep can result in the symptoms of a starvation even more dramatic than the symptoms caused by fasting from food. If sleeplessness is attempted for any prolonged period, our bodies may start failing in different ways.

Ten days of fasting from food has been tolerated by numbers of people. But ten days without sleep does not mean ten days of moderate discomfort, such as might be expected from a fast of this length. During these ten days, the most mentally alert may become confused, see imaginary objects and act insane. Even after these experimenters have had appropriate rest, it may be weeks before all their mental processes are restored to normal. Stories of short sleeping hours are well known in the cases of Churchill, Edison and Napoleon. Not so well known is the fact that daytime naps were part of the schedules of all these men, and a twenty-four hour record would usually show that they spent six to eight hours at rest.

The benefits of sleep are dramatically illustrated in the story of the humming bird. At the rate this tiny creature burns up energy when awake, it could only live two or three hours without food. However, during sleep, the humming bird's energy requirements are diminished to a point where it can sleep through the entire night without danger of starvation. When the humming bird sleeps, it enters a state of sleep far deeper than do humans. It can slow its energy requirements down greatly by nearly freezing during the night. This method of survival has been of interest to many scientists, particularly those interested in longevity.

Russian experimenters in the early fifties attempted to see what effect prolonged sleep could have on longevity. They used a fifteen year old dog, very near the end of its natural life span. Not only was it an old animal, it also showed signs of great age - falling hair, poor appetite, listless behavior. Through sedatives, and perhaps also the use of cold, this animal was put to sleep for ninety days. At the end of the period, it gained a new lease on life. It regained the vigor and hair of its middle years, and lived another six and one-half years. Death, when it came, was not from natural causes, but occurred during a fight with another animal.

This was a startling experiment, and its true meaning can be best understood by translating it into human terms. A dog, at fifteen years, is as old, in many ways, as a human at one hundred and twenty-five. Each - dog and man - have at that time lived to five times the age it took for their skeletons to mature. This is the length of time, from many scientific viewpoints, in which each is supposed to have lived his full life span. Adding the six and one-half years to the dog's life, then, would be equal to adding better than fifty-six years to a man's life - a grand total of one hundred eighty-one years. The only major drawback would be to find the old man who can be given this artificial sleep for about twenty-one years - for that would be the right proportion to the dog's ninety days, if we were to replicate this experiment with a human being.

How much a long sleep in the cold is worth may have also been demonstrated by the three groups known to have extremely long life spans in the world today. Both the Swiss and the Hunzingas live in mountainous territories where cold nights and a lack of heat are a regular part of their life. The other long-lived group may at first seem an enigma: the people who live in the Indian desert. However, deserts, though known for their great heat at mid-day, are barren of most plant life because of their cold at night. So, the people of

Rajasthan and other inhabitants of the desert also have a cold sleep every night. More work has to be done on the whole subject before more than speculation can be offered.

How much sleep do you need?

We were taught that eight hours sleep is considered the right and proper amount. It is a good average figure, but cannot be stated with absolute certainty to apply to each and every one of us at all times. We cannot point to various individuals who are getting along on less than eight hours and state with certainty that they are doing what is best for them. It is not hard to find numbers of doctors who feel strongly that too little sleep is frequently associated with a shortened life span. Nor, again, can we prove that great amounts of sleep lead to a much improved length of life - although there is that impression in the minds of many.

Six to nine hours' sleep is the amount of rest that most people need to feel refreshed and alert day after day. All of us have days when less than this is sufficient; and most of us also have days when quite a bit more would seem desirable. The problem of both sleep and its enemy, insomnia, will become far less troublesome when you are in good physical condition. Keeping your body in tune during the day will aid it to serve you better through all the twenty-four hours.

Sleeplessness is regarded with more concern than is usually justified. An occasional inability to fall into deep sleep is common with nearly everyone. Resting quietly in bed at such times can give us the minimum of relaxation and renewal we need for the next day. However, if such insomnia persists, it deserves to be called a habit rather than a disease. This pattern, frequent in older people, can be bothersome for all concerned. Chronic sleeplessness at night can result in a foggy, half-awake day, sure to be followed by another poor night. This vicious circle can be broken by making sure wakefulness is assured during the day. Add some definite, purposeful activity during the day-time hours. Prepare for a night's sleep by filling the day with action. Even a wide-awake day will not guarantee everyone a full night's sleep. Some individuals demand more than ordinary activity to enjoy complete rest.

If every bit of this advice has been tried, then it is time to seek medical help. There are diseases that can keep us from sleep, and the longer they are given the opportunity to exhaust us, the more seriously they may harm our health.

DREAMLAND *VERSUS* REALITY

Every night when our eyes close, we embark into the so-called dreamland. A place where anything and everything becomes a possibility; an interim border between fiction and perception; a place where the fabric of reality interwoven with the true essence of fantasy.

During each sleeping period, the body recharges and goes through a set of tasks to ensure it is at its best upon waking up. Memories are organized, re-organized and archived to provide the self with an updated reference index to interpret the upcoming reality.

Whilst awake, we live our days guided by our memories, which provide us with that referential index that makes electrical signals perceived by our sensory organs - what we call reality - to make sense. When the lights go off and we find ourselves sleeping, our memories and their interpretations are re-lived... and it does feel so real... only to realize it was "just a dream" when we wake up.

In real life, we find ourselves hand-in-hand with

whispers of memories which cause us, in many circumstances, to get stuck in the reference models as if they were the Holy Grail.

Whilst dreaming, we sometimes leave the unconscious state awaken and remember parts of the adventure. In the world of dreams, we can jump from memory to memory and experience them with such intensity, without even attempting to stop and consider their truthfulness. In having the possibility to jump and re-define our archived memories whilst dreaming we also have the option and the choice to redefine the content or the interconnection of each memory whilst awake…or whilst in an altered state also called meditative or hypnotic.

We constantly juggle memories to evaluate any and every situation we are involved in or with and automatically register new meanings as a result of the outcomes. As we do in dreams, we constantly swap this internal reference set of memories whilst being awake….and we do this unconsciously most of the time. We allow threads of information to raise stored memories to our internal reference screen all the time. Any bit of information that our brain captures from the external world is interpreted by our memory reference table so that we can give meaning to all that surrounds us. This is how we can find people we know in a crowded room – our brain is constantly analyzing the surroundings to get information that matches what we have already stored.

When these archived memories have a negative setting, we then have a recipe for disaster – there is a considerable possibility of projecting the same meanings to new situations as our brain establishes the necessary equivalences: we end up experiencing similar feelings and projecting these into upcoming events that have not yet happened. A clear example of this situation is the number one fear expressed by the American population – the fear of public speaking. A new occasion to speak in public may bring all the fears and stresses that can paralyze one's body even before this action is attempted.

Instead of freely creating and experiencing new events, we find ourselves imposing existing interpretations into upcoming events and clearly applying perception of reality as projections of archived memories. Day to day life stops being an adventure only to become a vicious cycle in which we continuously re-live our memories.

The border between dreamland and the so-called reality gets thinner and thinner. Whilst awake, we project our memories into the fabric of reality to interpret and to react to incoming stimuli and when sleeping, we project glimpses of reality into our dreams, which are, in fact, nothing more than our own "land of memories."

By default, we alter memories every time we bring them to our conscient screen, meaning every time we think about our archived memories, we color them with the new interpretations and conclusions of reality we have been acquiring – and this is why we find ourselves dumping belief systems we once considered *nothing but the truth*, such as "if we wish to speak up we need to raise our hand"… which was valid in kindergarten but no longer valid in an adult working environment where one needs to be proactive and charge forward, just like the earth that was once believed to be the centre of the Universe only to be discarded to second plan once the scientific community has accepted that fact.

By allowing stored memories not to be challenged and by not having a vigilant thinking mechanism in place to analyze and re-interpret events on the go, one is doomed to re-live the past, allocating for the present and upcoming future a reminiscence of the past, whatever this has been.

PART III

GETTING THE BEST OUT OF OUR BODIES
STRONGER BODY, STRONGER MIND
WALKING AND POSTURE
FITNESS REWARDS
UNOFFICIAL EXERCISES

STRONGER BODY, STRONGER MIND

To get started on a healthier, more enjoyable and longer life, we need to alter a few of our present habits. Most of us have developed these habits by accident and not as a result of careful planning. In the good old days before Cro-Magnon Man, this kind of accidental formation of habits was fine since one had to do strenuous work to eat, it did permit the most fit to survive. The demands on our bodies have become far less strenuous and the demands on our minds far greater than ever in the past. For example, in 1860 thirty per cent of the energy provided in the United States for building, logging and all other industries was supplied by muscle power. Today, less than one per cent of all the energy used in the United States is derived from man's muscles.

We must deliberately take care of our body if we are keen to have it functioning at its best. This has been shown in studies of undergraduates at West Point. Those that entered in good physical condition had the smallest number of emotional upsets and maintained the best average grades; those who just skimmed through on their fitness testing did poorly in their academic work and had a very high incidence of nervous breakdowns. The exercise we need does not have to be lengthy, nor does it require the purchase of expensive equipment. Five half-hours a week devoted to pleasant physical activities will bring us to the first step of prime physical fitness and keep us in top shape.

The benefits of such a program can be evaluated by its effect on only one symptom of life expectancy - blood pressure. Test after test has shown that even as little as a few months of this type of fitness activity increases the life span through dramatically reducing high blood pressure. If one now has high blood pressure, also called hypertension, one most certainly should consult a physician before beginning any exercise program.

Dietary needs must change for most of us if we are to avoid the early deaths of these times. Lumberjacks and construction workers can eat high fat diets and not get hardening of their arteries; sedentary workers - from bank presidents to file clerks - just don't burn up enough energy in their daily work to be protected from the high fat diet we all habitually eat. Physicians know that hardening of the arteries is related to deposits of fats within these arteries. Sedentary living and high fat diets are too often a fatal combination.

Redoing habits takes effort. How much depends largely on one's present habits. None of these changes are totally different from what we do now. They are more or less the addition and subtraction of a few habits in our total scheme of living.

In a survey made in 1954 G. Gallup sampled 29,000 Americans who had lived to be 100 or more and concluded that those who live longest are those who found a way to be healthy and to truly enjoy life.

How fit are we today?

A list of the various symptoms that arise from unfitness could be made into a fair-sized book. To get an introductory idea of one's present fitness state, ask the following questions:

- Are you "worn out" long before bedtime?
- Do your feet hurt day after day?
- Is your back a source of annoyance and pain?
- Do you mind standing when you have to wait for a moment, or do you immediately try to find a place to lean or sit?
- If you have to run for a train or cab, are you huffing for half an hour or do you shudder at the very thought?
- Do you think it would be possible for you to run up a flight of stairs today without strain?
- Are you bothered with stomach and bowel upsets?

- Do you have frequent headaches?
- Do you bounce out of bed in the morning or crawl out wishing you could sleep longer?
- Do you have trouble relaxing?
- Do you have trouble sleeping soundly at night?
- Do you suffer from frequent, unexplained tensions and a feeling of restlessness?

Strength, agility and endurance are all part of physical fitness. Many years ago, the health industry found that measuring the pulse rate before and after exercise was a good, quick, reliable method of estimating health in its relation to longevity. Over the years, this type of testing has been the object of much research and improvement:

- First, take your pulse while sitting at rest.
- Then hop fifty times, twenty-five hops on each foot.
- Take your pulse immediately after the last hop.
- Sit for two minutes, and then take your pulse again.

While you are hopping, an experienced observer could tell a great deal about your health simply by watching you. In fact, he could actually guess the pulse rate he will find at the end of the exercise. A normal pulse at rest - before the test - should be somewhere in between sixty and eighty-five beats per minute. Highly trained athletes may have a pulse lower than sixty; down to fifty or forty-eight is frequent. In the average person, though, a pulse as slow as that is more apt to indicate a heart problem than good physical condition.

After the test, an increase of the pulse up to an extra fifty beats per minute is considered satisfactory. Satisfactory in this instance means having what is now considered "normal" life expectancy. After the two-minute rest period, your pulse should have slowed down to about the rate first observed. Five or ten beats one way or the other are about the proper limits.

The healthier subject will usually show an actual reduction in his pulse rate after exercise. The untrained, dangerously out of condition man is the one who can't get his pulse rate down to even ten beats of its original rate.

Pulse rate	Normal results
Resting	60 – 85
Fifty hops	90 – 140
Two minutes rest	60 – 95

It is usually better to have someone else take your pulse, if possible. Not only will the examination be more accurate at rest this way, but a lot more meaningful after the exercise - when huffing, to take your own pulse may become a considerable challenge.

If you have difficulty knowing how to take a pulse, a

few words may help you, or your associate, in discovering where it is, and what messages it is sending. Most people have their pulse beat located on the side of the wrist near the thumb. In some individuals, however, it may be located on the top of the wrist or on the side near the little finger. In feeling for the pulse, never use your thumb, since it has its own pulse, and you will find these beats confusing and adding to the pulse rate at the wrist.

There are times one cannot find a pulse at the wrist. Either the artery lies too deep to give a perceptible impulse, or the artery has spread out into several small branches. If this is the case, the best advice is to look for a good pulse elsewhere. The neck is the best place to find a pulse in a fairly constant location. Place your three fingers together on your neck at a position midway between a line drawn down from the ear and center of the neck. You will undoubtedly feel some sort of pulsation. Slowly, and without too much pressure, move your fingers from this point either to the center of the neck, or back to the ear. Exploring in this manner will quickly show you where the strongest point of pulsation occurs. Once you have found the pulse in your own neck you will be able to find it readily in another person.

A healthy pulse has a good bounce and will keep on with its regular rhythm even as it is put under moderate finger pressure. If you find a pulse that seems more like a little pipe, hard and lumpy, you may have a hardened artery. Although this is not the same type of hardened artery associated with heart failure, it is a sufficient warning to stop further pulse testing and seek medical attention.

The pulse also may seem small. Physicians usually use the term, *thready*. As you might suspect, such an unusually small pulse represents a heart that is not pumping a full, adequate supply of blood to the body. Once again, go to your doctor and get his advice.

Any pulse that is not giving a regular rhythmic beat is also to be suspected. Fortunately irregular pulses are rare, but if you find a rate that does not read out like 1-1-1-1 it would be wise to consult your physician.

Abnormal pulses may read: 1—1,2-1,1,1---- 1,2, or 1,1,1—1. This type of test is an excellent starting place. It can serve as a speedy reassurance for those in fair to good condition, and as a real warning to those too far out of condition. If you can't pass this test, your exercise program must start out more slowly than would otherwise be advisable.

Too many of today's successful men and women have gained their positions of prominence through hard mental work and self-control. If these same people leap with full force into an exercise program, they will misinterpret the term "vigorous" to their own disadvantage. Knowing from previous experience vigor in mental activities, they may expect their bodies to be capable of as much strain as their mentalities, therefore, you should adapt your exercise program to the results of this test in this way: even if the resting pulse is over 85, but under 95, it is still safe to go ahead with the test. However, if any signs of strain, shortness of breath, chest discomfort or dizziness appear during the hops, stop immediately and check pulse.

As long as your pulse remains below 150, there is no need for concern. This indicates, usually, too much weight and too little physical reserve. In the specific exercises to follow, rope skipping should be avoided until this test can be passed, and the walking program should be restricted to a maximum of fast walking - no trotting. If, however, the resting pulse does not return to five or ten points within the two-minute interval, keep on checking it at two-minute intervals. If it has returned to normal by four minutes there is no need for alarm, but the need of a fitness program is even more definite.

At six minutes the pulse rate had better be down to normal limits if you wish to carry out any plans of more extenuous exercise. Though this pulse test is a good benchmark it will not do to show real fitness, nor can it serve to show one's progress in an objective and meaningful manner. For those objectives, we must turn to the second test.

The test chosen to help us in this progress objective is a real endurance test. This second test is known as the Seventeen-Inch Bench-Step Test and has been extensively researched and standardized by the US Air Force. It can be done with a minimum of training equipment whilst giving relative accurate results.

A bench that measures exactly seventeen inches in height need not be purchased - nearly any sturdy chair in the house can be put into service. Its basic requirement is that of stability and strength; in doing the test, this chair or bench is going to be carrying all your weight - Its height does not have to be an exact seventeen inches to get reasonable accurate results in your tests; any height between fifteen and eighteen inches will serve sufficiently well.

Since the technique of the test demands that you step up on the chair first with one foot, then with the other, your own height should have some consideration in selecting a proper height surface for stepping. A woman five feet tall is going to work very hard stepping up seventeen inches, and a six-foot six man may not be working hard enough by only raising himself up the same seventeen inches.

To achieve the best results, this test should be done two or three hours after a meal, and only when you are feeling reasonably well. A slight cold or even a mild headache will just get worse during the test and fail to give a correct estimate of your fitness. You also don't need a new outfit of gym clothes, and clothing should be kept at a minimum.

It makes no difference which foot you begin the test with, but for the purpose of description we will follow the ancient tradition and start with the left foot:

- Take, or have someone else take your pulse. Stand next to the chair.
- Raise your left foot up on the chair quickly.
- Raise your body up on the chair by placing your right foot on the chair.
- Bring your left foot down.
- And then bring your right foot down.

As you do this, if you can find sufficient breath, count 1, 2, 3, and 4 in sequence with the four different steps. This will give you timing and rhythm and will prevent you from slowing down in going through this set of tests. Do this exercise at a rate of thirty times a minute. We are examining for endurance, not for strength.

The following chart illustrates the results typically obtained during this test:

	Stepping	Pulse	Rates
	Time	Men	Women
Beginning	30 seconds	100 or less	110 or less
Intermediate	1 minute	100 or less	110 or less
Advanced	2 minutes	100 or less	110 or less
Energetic	3 minutes	140 or less	150 or less
Dynamic	5 minutes	150 or less	160 or less

Repeat this sequence the number of times shown on the chart above: start with the beginner's 30-second test and increasing the time until your pulse rate exceeds 100 beats per minute. At the end of the test sit and rest for one minute, then have your pulse rate checked, beginning at the second minute of rest.

Above all, don't be discouraged by your performance: these final two sections may never be within your range of accomplishment; they are performance standards that athletes aim for. The closer you come to attaining this degree of fitness, the more you are doing to assure yourself of the healthy added years you envisage.

Review your recent use of time with the following questionnaire and find where to slip these thirty-minute sessions in your day.

Fitness questionnaire

Honestly and accurately recall where you were yesterday. Search for a half hour, three times a week that won't be missed. It does not have to be the same half-hour each day:

Weekends
- At what time do you get up each morning on Saturday? And on Sunday?
- When you got up did you feel refreshed?
- Did you have breakfast immediately—or would you welcome a half-hour exercise period to really wake you up?

- Can you fit at least one half-hour exercise period on weekends?

Working days
- How many coffee and rest breaks do you take each working day?
- What do you do with these breaks?
- How long is your lunch period? How do you use this time?
- Can you get in one exercise period per week during lunch time or in the afternoon?

Leaving work
- At what time do you leave work?

- How tired do you feel when you get home?
- How did you spend the evening?
- What time do you go to bed?
- Can you get in one exercise period per week before bedtime to help you sleep better?

We learn to walk by imitation. Most of those whom we imitated were probably too tired to care, either how they stood or how they walked and, certainly, they did not realize that they were acting as examples.

We grew up walking with their slumped shoulders, their protruding stomach and all their fatigue, sore feet, and aching backs. Now we have to learn to walk all over again - the right way. It's easy; it uses far less energy and it pays big dividends in comfort and strength. Before walking correctly we must stand correctly. Then as we walk we will find out that by having our standing posture correct, our walking posture will be easier and more natural.

It is easy to learn to stand the right way: stand up against a wall then simply flatten the small curve of your back against that wall. What happens? Your pelvis goes toward the wall at the top, and comes out, away from the wall at the bottom. Your tail is tucked away toward the back of your legs and your tummy goes in. You feel thinner immediately, and you show it. To do this muscle movement correctly, you must keep your knees locked and your heels touching the wall throughout the exercise. After you have achieved the proper stance, tighten up all the muscles that you are using to hold it. Now hold them for six seconds, and relax. This posture exercise can be done in the same fashion, at the same time, as the other isometric exercises; if you need strength for correct posture, as most of us do, it will perform wonders in a few short weeks.

"Lift up your feet, when walking" is a tip many of us have heard but few have put into practice. Yet this is an essential part of the correct method of walking. Most of us push one foot along the ground, while we slide the other foot into a position for a new push. The posture exercise, while standing at the wall, is the beginning of good walking. To take a first step towards this new walk, don't push away from that wall; instead, slightly lift up your leg from the thigh. Move it upward and forward, and then put it down. Then lift up the other leg from the thigh, and put it down. This is good walking. It may help to lift up your leg if you concentrate on the muscles in the front of your leg from your pelvis to your knee. These are the ones that do the lifting. Now, walk around the room two or three times this new way and come back to the wall. You may find that your back is much flatter than when you first stood at that wall. Or, to say it another way, your posture - both standing and walking - is straighter. To get the most grace and comfort in your new walking you should make sure that your knees nearly touch as they pass each other. Also, look at your toes as you walk. The more nearly you can keep them pointed straight ahead, the better your walk will be. Check your shoes. An even slightly run-down heel on your shoe can keep you from straightening out your foot to the desired straight-ahead direction.

A commonly recommended exercise for weak or sore feet is to pick up your socks from the floor with your bare feet several times each day. A little practice and a little time out of hard-soled shoes will make the toes sufficiently flexible to accomplish this task. Another method is to pick a marble off the floor with your toes. This will also exercise the rest of the muscles in your feet.

Many of us walk all day long with our toes in an almost paralyzed position. The more flexibility we develop in our feet the more comfort we will have in walking - and even running will become enjoyable instead of being a painful task. There is even a slight economic advantage to this style of walking: the heels on your shoes won't wear out nearly so fast! Since you are lifting, not pushing your foot, it comes down flat on the ground, very little weight is placed on your heel. The ball of your foot will begin to come alive, and your toes will feel more active than they have been for years. The rest of your posture will automatically take care of itself.

Chin in, chest out, etc. Much more important, you will want to start that program of regular daily walking that you know you must begin.

Spinal Health

Doing things the wrong way seems to come naturally to most of us. We have been given bad examples from our childhood days. Many of us know how to use our backs correctly; yet we can't be bothered to put this knowledge to good use when we pick up or carry something. There may even be group ridicule for anyone who decides to use his back correctly.

These problems of the correct use of the back are not confined to the occasional individual who does heavy manual labor; they are common to all of us: the housewife, standing at a sink, or picking up her baby, exposes her back to as many hazards as does the construction laborer. She may even incur in greater danger, for she has less to help her in the way of machinery. Also, her husband, with his enforced hobbies of lawn care, may really know less about taking care of his back than any foreman would tolerate for his workers. The commonest causes of financial loss to employers and insurance companies are back problems, many of which are preventable.

"The possession of physical strength, agility and endurance may enable the individual to survive, while the lack of fitness may spell catastrophe". These words expressed the thoughtful opinion of the American Medical Association and the American Association for Health, Physical Education and Recreation in 1958, on the prime value of fitness: survival. But what about the other advantages of being fit? What good is it to live a long life, unless you have the health, strength, vitality, vigor and virility you want? The statement of the doctors and physical educators does not stop at mere comments concerning the relation of fitness and long life.

Prolonged inactivity, they say, is marked by a decline in the efficiency of both our hearts and our lungs. This is the same story that the rest of life teaches us: no resting on the oars. You must either swim upstream, towards safety, or drift downstream towards disaster. This joint statement of the American Medical Association and the American Association for Health, Physical Education and Recreation also adverts that as we engage in a fitness program, our heart and circulatory system will be trained to become far more efficient. This efficiency will be demonstrated in more economical pumping action of the heart, throughout the entire body. And not only will our heart and blood vessels work better, our lungs will also increase in efficiency.

There is currently no evidence that physical fitness can grow hair for the bald, but it will help to maintain what hair you have through better circulation - and perhaps through the increased attention you give your entire body. Your blood vessels, especially your arteries, are going to get bigger and better. Various studies have shown that the arteries of physically active people are up to four or five times larger than the arteries of the sitters. At least as important is the equally well demonstrated fact that one will grow new blood vessels and provide the body with better overall circulation. Adding improved posture and strength to this equation will allow the internal organs to function in a more optimized manner.

Our body was conceived with a correct place for every organ. Years of faulty posture have pushed and pulled many people's internal architecture into new, surrealistic arrangements that don't work as well as the original setting. The commonest symptom of this displacement is that of bowel upsets. In women, furthermore, menstrual disorders also occur.

Experimental evidence has shown that a program of fitness can reduce these functional disorders that are becoming more and more common. Bowel upsets, constipation and menstrual disorders have all been shown to benefit from a regular program of exercise. Whilst observing people in the street one sees that many do not walk - instead, slouch along. They don't stand, they lean - or tilt; their skin portrays signs of internal struggle or below optimum overall body performance.

Action, participation and recognition are what society teaches us to aim for. As we develop our bodies, we will find our energies more responsive and more dependable. Your skin will acquire a glow previously unknown and this comes from a new exposure to elements from an appropriate nutrition, exercise and relaxation program. The activity experienced by your skin whilst practicing any form of exercise or outdoor activities act as a far finer balm than any to be found on cosmetic shelves. These are not the only benefits of a sound, fit body; your mental stamina and resilience will also improve in direct proportion to the attainment of your fitness goals.

A sound mind in a sound body is not the most appropriate way of expressing this truth. We are not made up of parts; each of us is an organic unit. We think, feel and reason with the section of this unit called the brain. It needs a good supply of blood and other nourishment to carry out its functions. Those who are fit already know, apparently as a delightful secret, that fitness will greatly improve sexual vigor. Men have fathered children when they were ninety years of age. On the other hand, sexual activity, as it involves great muscular work, can be a disastrous overload for one out of condition. Certainly, some heart attacks are related to the sudden efforts of love-making and can surely be minimized by following an ongoing fitness routine.

The too frequent mental lapses of the aged are often due to insufficient circulation of blood through their brain. Such lapses may appear to be overnight disasters, but they rarely are. Usually a lack of circulation has been caused by years of continuous sitting, by overeating, and by other habits of a lifetime devoted to unfitness.

Last, adding to all these benefits, your disposition must improve - it has no choice. "Rush, rush - time is running out," can sound quite real if you look at the mortality tables and hope for average luck. But that same cry of woe loses much of its urgency when you look at it from the perspective of a life only half lived at fifty; with the best - freedom, health and wisdom - yet to be savored after ninety.

In Sweden, as previously mentioned, the coffee break has been frequently replaced by the exercise break. Some examples of these stand-up, quick, easy-to-do exercises are given below. Another country, Russia, has also adopted these rest-break exercises with a strong affirmative.

The so-called quiet (or "unofficial") exercises are add-ons to any ongoing fitness program, as the first steps of an exercise-commitment. These can be done while attending a meeting or when going to the water cooler and are as simple as tensing selected muscles for a brief moment and subsequently relaxing them; one can make the muscles of one's left leg tight for a moment, and then let these muscles go limp whist tensing the muscles of one's right leg. This can be done while standing or sitting.

Quiet exercises, walking and running can be the major physical activities to maintain excellent health. They can be an equally powerful weapon in one's armory of fitness. Exercise should not only be made respectable, but part of our daily life, almost like brushing our teeth and bathing, yet few of us think of exercise in the same way. We should learn to think of fitness as being at least as much a part of our daily grooming as are the other parts of our health rituals. Why not adapt the Swedish exercise break to one's own office routine? Why not substitute such an exercise break for the gossip and coffee sessions? The exercises are all comfortable and require no special equipment or dress-up code for full participation. For many reasons, there are no push-ups, pull-ups, knee-bends or other outmoded styles of mock heroic activities. All of these movements are done in almost any position, and involve mainly the trunk and arms.

A description of eight work-break activities is included below. Morale, vitality and efficiency, as well as longevity, will be the ultimate reward.

Exercise 1
Stand up. Place your hands on your hips and rotate your head, shoulders and upper trunk as a unit in a slight circle. Do this eight times.

Exercise 2
Swing your right hand and arm in an up-and-down circle at the side of your body. Do this five times. Then do the same exercise with your left arm.

Exercise 3

With your arms against your waist, alternately kick out to 15 or 20 degrees, first with your left, then with your right leg. Do this ten to twenty times.

Exercise 4

While standing, bring your hands in front of your body and bend down to touch some part of your legs between your knees and your ankles. Do this five times.

Exercise 5

While standing with your arms straight at your sides, rotate your head in a circle trying to touch your shoulders with your ears. Make a full circle five times in each clockwise and anti-clockwise direction.

Exercise 6

Place your hands at your sides and roll your shoulders about their center five times.

Exercise 7

While standing, place your hands in front with your fingers gripping imaginary oars. Bring your hands diagonally up to your shoulders in a rowing motion. This can be done five to ten times.

Exercise 8

Stand on your toes and reach for the ceiling with your arms. Pause a moment, then come back down on your feet. Do this five times.

All these exercises can be done in ordinary clothes and in conventional postures; no special equipment is needed, nor is a great deal of extra space necessary.

Breathing exercises

Breathing exercises have been in and out of vogue since the early 1800's. They can serve as an excellent non-caloric form of refreshment as well as giving our muscles some much needed motion.

Exercise 1

Sit on a chair with your feet about nine inches apart. Lean forward and hold the front legs of the chair. In this position inhale and exhale deeply. Repeat 3 – 4 times and then rest. Since this position fixes the muscles of the shoulders, all the breathing effort will be done by the abdominal musculature.

Exercise 2

Lean back in an armchair and press your shoulders against it. Stretch your feet out in front on a hassock or footrest. Again, take three or four deep breaths for this exercise, and rest.

The so-called unofficial exercise program outlined in the previous paragraphs is a minimum fitness schedule. Most of us can do more. Sports bring us out of doors and give us a variety of physical activity that prevents boredom. They also give our minds new challenges with attendant pleasure at their solution.

After a period of difficult work, the change to satisfying sports can do far more to reboot our system than any number of hours of sleep, or of passing time watching the activities of others in a ball park or on a TV screen. Certainly the easiest way to get out of doors is to go for a walk or, if you leave close to nature, hiking. You can participate in this wonderfully beneficial sport in your own neighborhood. The equipment needed for walking and hiking can be bought for a surprisingly low price, and will return its cost many times over in the comfort it brings.

A good pair of shoes certainly is first on the list and since shoes should be worn with a pair of heavy socks, they should be fitted over the socks. A composition sole with a pattern is best to give good footing when in the woods. High shoes and boots are not comfortable to wear on most hiking tours, as they bend and chafe the leg and cut off ventilation. The rest of the clothing should be a combination of personal taste, personal budget, and geography. A lightweight cotton windbreaker, sufficiently inconspicuous on warm days, can also give real protection from sudden rains and chilling winds. A woolen shirt of appropriate weight is probably the most all-around useful item that any hiker can have for any but the hottest days. Good wool will have a surprising degree of water resistance and warmth. Loose trousers for men, slacks for women, are the most useful leg garments. Any tightly-fitted garment will bind and turn a hike into an endurance contest.

As side equipment, a canteen or plastic bottle for water is always handy to have on a hike - even if no cooking is planned. Thirst is an unpleasant sensation that can grow into quite a problem when no relief is available. In fact, many years ago, with much planning and the help of every conceivable expert, one stratospheric balloonist almost proved with his life that water is a valuable asset. During the night prior to the ascent, this man, busy with preparations, did not drink any liquids. As the flight began, he became thirsty, but since no water had been provided, he completed the flight with far more courage than comfort. At the time of his descent, his fever was so high that there was real alarm for his life. He barely survived.

The hiker's problems are far less severe than the

balloonist's but to most of us they can seem equally bad when we want the simplest of life's requirements and find they are not there to be had.

Camping, the next step up from hiking is an inexpensive method of sightseeing, and a nice way to become acquainted with many fine people that you would not meet in any other way. In the case of camping equipment, a happy solution can be found in the many fine stores that rent such equipment. By trial and error, and following good advice from these stores, it is possible to find what is necessary for one's concept of hiking and camping.

Although most of us can go for some sort of hike in the woods, less of us are able to go for swimming, sailing, skiing and other elite sports. Those who are able to engage in these recreational opportunities - and fortunately the number of aficionados on these type of activities is growing every year - should use them as a means of increasing one's fitness and one's enjoyment of life.

Not all recreation must contribute to fitness, of course, but why shouldn't we get as much fitness out of our recreation as humanly possible? Playing a different sport each season will add to fun and companionship. Our bodies will gain a new vitality through exposure to the weather - a glow and vigor they can never acquire in the protection of controlled warmth during winter and air conditioning in summer. Our cars must be tuned up at regular intervals and most of them need to be given a fairly good high speed run at times, to keep from getting all stuck up with carbon and gum. Yet the idea of a good high speed walk, even a moderately uncomfortable one, seems out of the question for most of us. The following research findings, presented in the publication *Physical Fitness for Adults* should be taken seriously by those who are interested in a healthy life: "that (1) a sound heart cannot be damaged by exercise; (2) that more heart and circulatory troubles result from too mild and too short exercise periods; and (3) that exercise is needed to normalize the blood chemistry in the face of higher fat consumption in modern diets."

PART IV

NUTRITION: HEALTHIER CHOICES
PLANT-BASED FOOD
VEGETABLES AND FRUITS: 5+ A DAY
FOOD-BIOAVAILABILITY & WATER
A QUICK WORD ON DIETS

PLANT-BASED FOOD

Vegetables and fruits have been an essential part of human diet since the dawn of mankind. Juiced or dehydrated leaves from cereal grasses only started to be included in the human diet in the last century. Since then, a great amount of literature has been published, providing information on their composition and the benefits for which they may be responsible, along with other studies on the use of vegetables and fruits.

Although it is beyond the scope of this chapter to provide a detailed description of all the advantages vegetables and cereal grasses – green food - as well as fruits, account for in terms of human health, the information presented is far from being exhaustive. It only caters for key highlights on the research performed throughout the years on this topic, including the increasing awareness and understanding of its positive impact in global health by helping preventing chronic diseases that stem from unbalanced and unhealthy diets.

Cereal grasses

The consumption of wheatgrass in the Western world started in the 1930s, as Charles F. Schnabel, an agricultural chemist from Kansas City, discovered the nutritional advantages of a diet including young cereal grasses for both animal and human consumption. By that time, cereal grass and the so called "Grass Juice Factor", a water soluble extract from grass juice, was intensely studied. G. Kohler and co-researchers, at the University of Wisconsin, began investigating the reasons behind the higher nutritional value of the summer milk in the diet of rats and guinea pigs. They concluded that the grasses eaten by the cows that provided the milk, during spring and summer, was the key factor behind the improved nutritional value of the milk; M. Cannon and colleagues, at the University of California, Berkeley, found that the addition of dehydrated grass or grass juice to the stock ration of guinea pigs induced remarkable recovery and re-stimulated their growth, whilst Graham and colleagues studied the nutritional properties of cereal grasses and suggested their use as a human food supplement, as a cost-effective way to provide important nutrients, like vitamins, minerals and proteins, frequently lacking in the American and in many world-wide diets.

The "health factor" in cereal grasses was studied through the 1940s and 1950s and found to have different health-related effects on animals, such as blocking the development of vitamin C deficiency, sustaining the growth of several beneficial intestinal bacteria and promoting the healing of peptic ulcers, among many other benefits.

During the 1960s and 1970s, there were great social changes and environmental awareness increased drastically around the world. The attention on "natural foods and therapies" started to grow rapidly. Anne Wigmore studied and "re-discovered" the benefits of wheat grass and wheat grass juice, considered as a diet complement for humans and, in 1968, she founded the Hippocrates Health Institute (HHI) in Boston.

This "superfood" became a well known health and diet food, providing optimal health and exhibiting healing properties. Wigmore started treating her guests with chronic degenerative diseases by using wheatgrass and wheatgrass juice therapies, along with a diet of green and raw foods. Many guests at HHI claimed to be cured from diseases deemed incurable by their physicians, after being submitted to the simple therapy based on wheatgrass.

In Japan, research pharmacist Y. Hagiwara began studying the benefits of diets based on cereal grasses at about the same time Wigmore started working at HHI. As Schnabel did some fifty decades earlier, he found that "the leaves of the cereal grasses provide the nearest thing to the perfect food that this planet offers". He also carried out several animal and human experiments with colleagues in America and Japan to evaluate the health benefits of different cereal grass juices, and found that grasses of wheat, oats, rye and barley were remarkably high in many nutrients.

Other Japanese researchers have focused their studies mainly on barley grass, although no significant nutrient differences were found between cereal grasses. These studies, as those performed on wheat grass, also suggest various beneficial uses for barley grass juice. A "plant factor" was identified in grasses, as well as in alfalfa and broccoli, providing significant growth stimulation when fed to guinea pigs, and a potent anti-inflammatory protein was isolated from barley leaves; the positive effects of treating skin diseases and ulcers with barley grass juice was suggested, and the effects of that juice on the endurance and motor activity in mice was reported. Further studies indicate that supplementation with barley leaves may help to scavenge oxygen free radicals, save the LDL-vitamin E content and inhibit LDL oxidation; moreover, the addition of vitamins C and E to barley leaves can inhibit the Sd-LDL oxidation more effectively, which may protect against vascular diseases in type 2 diabetic patients. Other experiments suggest the importance of the antioxidant and hypolipidemic properties of barley leaves essence in the prevention of cardiovascular disease, such as atherosclerosis.

Green Food and Fruits

New studies performed during the 1970s, the 1980s and the 1990s by researchers continue to suggest the benefits of "green foods". Among them are those indicating that chlorophyll in wheat sprout extract inhibits the metabolic activation of carcinogens *in vitro*, and those connecting several green vegetables to anti-mutagenic protection; other studies link a significant decrease in the incidence of cancer in mice to a special diet consisting of wheat grass, carrots, several fruits and sunflower seeds, supplemented with high doses of vitamin C. These studies on this topic also suggest the lower risk of appendicitis upon consumption of vegetables, mainly green vegetables.

In 1996, Steinmetz and collaborators published a review of the scientific literature on the relationship between vegetable and fruit consumption and the risk of cancer, gathering results from 206 human epidemiologic studies and 22 animal studies. The evidence for a protective effect of greater vegetable and fruit consumption is consistent for cancers of stomach, esophagus, lung, oral cavity and pharynx, endometrium, pancreas and colon. The types of vegetables or fruit that most often appear to be protective against cancer are raw vegetables, followed by allium vegetables, carrots, green vegetables, cruciferous vegetables, and tomatoes. Substances present in vegetables and fruit that may help to protect against cancer and their mechanisms include dithiolthiones, isothiocyanates, indole-3-carbinol, allium compounds, isoflavones, protease inhibitors, saponins, phytosterols, inositol hexaphosphate, vitamin C, D-limonene, lutein, folic acid, beta carotene, lycopene, selenium, vitamin E, flavonoids, and dietary fiber. Other effects of increased vegetable and fruit consumption also aid the human body in the fight against cardiovascular disease, diabetes, stroke, obesity, diverticulitis and cataracts. Additional research by the end of the 20th century suggests that uncooked, lactobacilli-rich, vegan food decreases subjective symptoms of rheumatoid, and that people who consumed a substantial amount of green vegetables may have a reduced risk of colon cancer.

Investigations on this theme are still part of the syllabus of research of reputed laboratories all around the world, aiming to clarify the real benefits of cereal grasses, green vegetables, fruits and other raw nutrients in the human diet.

Studies on the effect of regular intake of wheat grass

juice suggest that this therapy may be effective and safe as a single or adjuvant treatment of active distal ulcerative colitis and that it also has potential to decrease the need for blood transfusion in children with thalassemia major. A reduction in the need for blood and bone marrow building medications during chemotherapy in breast cancer patients was also related as a possible benefit of wheat grass juice intake, without diminishing the effects of the therapy.

Further research suggests that the impact of nutrition on obstructive lung disease is most evident for antioxidant vitamins, particularly vitamin C and, to a lesser extent, vitamin E; moreover, components of raw vegetables and some micronutrients appear to decrease breast cancer risk, and both raw and cooked vegetable consumption are inversely related to epithelial cancers, particularly those of the upper gastrointestinal tract and possibly breast cancer. These relationships may be even stronger for a primarily raw vegetable diet.

A cross-sectional study performed on meat-eating, vegetarian, and vegan men in the United Kingdom suggest that when animal foods are excluded from the diet, the endogenous production of EPA and DHA results in low but stable plasma concentrations of these fatty acids. Other studies relate diets high in natural chlorophyll (but not chlorophyllin, a semi synthetic derivative of chlorophyll present in higher concentrations in green leafy vegetables) to lower rates of colon cancer - chlorophylls and carotenoids may in part explain the widely accepted protective effects of green vegetable consumption against cancer. In addition, intakes of reduced dietary fat and increased fiber, vegetable, fruit and other nutrients may improve overall survival in postmenopausal women diagnosed with breast cancer, while increased intake of some fruits, vegetables and soy foods may be associated with breast cancer risk reduction in Korean women, as well as in Chinese women.

Finally, a 2011 cross-sectional analysis of 1999 - 2004 data from US National Health and Nutrition Examination Survey suggests that vegetarian diets are nutrient dense, consistent with dietary guidelines, and could be recommended for weight management without compromising diet quality.

Old claims for the health properties of cereal grass diets, ranging from promotion of general well-being to cancer prevention has not still been totally corroborated in the scientific literature and to this date, the so-called "Grass Juice Factor" in young green plants has still not been identified.

However, recent research data arising from pilot studies with small samples support the beneficial effects of chlorophyll in the human diet and deeper investigation is currently being performed to substantiate the scientific evidence.

Nutrients in "green food" and fruits

Doctors, nutritionists as well as health and government agencies generally recommend a daily intake of, at least, 2 - 5 servings of vegetables and/or fruits, depending on gender, age and physical activity levels. In fact, vegetables, fruits and cereal grasses are major contributors of a number of nutrients that are frequently neglected by humans. They are a source of macronutrients, such as carbohydrates (e.g. starch, sugars and fiber), fats (e.g. unsaturated fats), proteins and water, as well as micronutrients, such as minerals (e.g. calcium, iron, magnesium and potassium) and vitamins (e.g. A, B_2, B_6, Folate, C, E and K). Their consumption is associated with a reduced risk of many chronic diseases and evidence indicates that the intake of vegetables and fruits is important in the prevention of cardiovascular diseases, including heart attack and stroke. Moreover, most vegetables and fruits (as well as cereal grasses), when prepared without added fats or sugars, are relatively low in calories. Eating them instead of higher caloric foods can help adults and children achieve and maintain a healthy weight.

Fiber

Dietary fiber, also known as bulk or roughage, consists of all parts of plant foods that the human body cannot digest or absorb, thus passing relatively intact through the stomach, small intestine, colon and out of the body.

Fiber is commonly classified into insoluble and soluble. Insoluble fiber does not dissolve in water and may only be fermented, to a limited extent, in the colon. It promotes the movement of ingested foods through the digestive tract, increasing stool bulk. Soluble fiber dissolves in water and is readily fermented in the colon into gases and physiologically active byproducts.

The best known benefit of dietary fiber in humans is to prevent or reduce constipation. Several studies performed on this constituent indicate several other important advantages associated with its consumption; dietary fiber intake may reduce cancer and a high intake, particularly of its soluble type, improves glycemic control, decreases hyperinsulinemia and lowers plasma lipid concentrations in patients with type 2 diabetes. Furthermore, increased fiber intake also benefits a number of gastrointestinal disorders, including gastroesophageal reflux disease, duodenal ulcer, diverticulitis, constipation and hemorrhoids. High fiber and fruit intakes is also associated with a decrease in Crohn's disease risk, while high vegetable intake is related with decreased in ulcerative colitis risk.

Soluble fiber is found in all plants in varying quantities, whereas insoluble fiber may be obtained from vegetables such as green beans, celery, cauliflower, zucchini, cereal grasses, from fruits, such as avocado and bananas, as well as from whole grains, such as seeds and nuts. The amount of each type of fiber varies in different foods and so, to receive the greatest health benefit, a wide variety of high-fiber foods should be included in the diets.

Proteins

Proteins are complex organic compounds that make up most of the body's weight, just second to water. Their basic structure is a chain of amino acids, which can combine in numerous ways, each being responsible for a specific function. When a protein food is ingested, the body breaks it down into amino acids through digestion, involving typically the action of enzymes called proteases. Healthy adult humans can make in adequate quantities all but nine of the needed amino acids - the so-called essential amino acids - that must be obtained from daily food intakes.

Every cell in the human body contains proteins, which are of primary importance in the growth and development of all body tissues, being the building material for these different tissues, such as nails, hair, skin, blood and for muscles and internal organs, such as the heart and the brain. They are also a component of hormones and enzymes which are responsible for numerous body functions, such as water balance and prevention of blood and tissues from becoming either too acid or too alkaline. Moreover, the constituent amino acids of proteins act as precursors of many coenzymes, hormones, nucleic acids, and other molecules essential for life.

Protein from animal sources, such as meat, fish, poultry, eggs and dairy products, is often called complete, because it contains all the essential amino acids. Vegetable protein sources, such as beans, peas, nuts, seeds, and grain are considered by today's experts in this field as incomplete as they lack one or more of those essential amino acids, with the exception made for soybean which is a source of all essential amino acids.

From a vegetarian perspective, a diet including a wide variety of protein-rich vegetable foods may also supply all essential amino acids. Combining beans with brown rice, corn, nuts, seeds or wheat is a way of obtaining all essential amino acids. Further studies indicate that protein found in green leafy plants is relatively consistent in nature and that protein in cereal grass is superior to that of other plant and animal sources.

Vitamins

Vitamins are organic compounds that are essential for the normal growth of multicelular organisms and are needed in very small amounts. Several vitamins have been identified, some of which are water-soluble (as those from the B complex and vitamin C) whilst others are fat-soluble (vitamins A, D, E and K). Water soluble vitamins, in general, dissolve easily in water, and are readily excreted from the body through the urine, which is a good predictor of vitamin consumption. The fat-soluble vitamins are absorbed in the intestinal tract with the help of fats and can be stored in the body.

In humans, most vitamins can be supplied by plant-based foods except for vitamins D, synthesized in the skin with the help of ultraviolet radiation from the sun, and B_{12}, generally considered to be absent in plant foods, although some reports indicate it as a component of cereal grasses. Vitamin B_{12} found in wheat and barley grasses may be there in connection with microbes from the soils in which the grasses are grown, or lactobacilli which are known to be present on cereal grasses.

Vitamin A

Vitamin A, a fat soluble vitamin, includes (among others) retinol, pre-formed vitamin A naturally present in foods of animal origin, namely fish, dairy products and liver, and pro-vitamin A, carotenoids present in vegetables, fruits and oils, which are transformed in vitamin A in the body. Plant carotenoids are the primary dietary source of pro-vitamin A worldwide, with β-carotene as the most well-known pro-vitamin A carotenoid. The excessive intake of this carotenoid may induce carotenodermia, a harmless condition detected by the body's skin presenting an orange-like tint arising from deposition of this compound in the epidermis.

Among other functions, this vitamin is important for vision, supports production of anti-bodies, enhances the immune response of polymorphonuclear leukocytes and other white blood cells, assists in the synthesis of DNA and RNA and, like vitamins E, C and β-carotene, is an important anti-oxidant, reducing free radicals, which are thought to cause cell aging and, in some cases, cancer; furthermore, both vitamin A and carotene have been demonstrated to reduce the risk of certain cancers, particularly those of epithelial tissues – skin, lung and cervical cancers.

β-carotene is present in yellow/orange vegetables like carrots, fruits like cantaloupe, mango, papaya and squash, as well as in leafy greens, such as kale, spinach, broccoli and cereal grasses.

Vitamin B6

Vitamin B6 is a water-soluble vitamin that includes a group of six related compounds, pyridoxine (PN), pyridoxal (PL) and pyridoxamine (PM) plus their respective phosphates – PNP, PLP and PMP. In animal tissues, PLP and PMP are the most common forms found, while PN and PNP are the mostly found in plant foods. Vitamin B6 is involved in many aspects of macronutrient metabolism, in the synthesis of neurotransmitters and histamine, as well as in the synthesis and function of hemoglobin and gene expression. PLP also serves as a coenzyme for many reactions.

Besides animal sources, vitamin B6 can be found in many plant foods, including green leafy vegetables (e.g. spinach), tomato, potato, garbanzo beans, lima beans, soybeans, in fruits like banana and avocado as well as in some nuts and seeds. Cereal grasses are also indicated as a good source of pyridoxine.

Folate

Folate is a water-soluble B-vitamin occurring naturally in food. Its synthetic form is folic acid. This vitamin is involved in the duplication of chromosomes during cell reproduction, preventing birth abnormalities and mental disorders, as well as in the synthesis of specific proteins, such as hemoglobin, preventing anemia. It also acts as an intermediary in biochemical reactions involving the transfer of a single carbon atom between two substances and regulates blood homocysteine levels, an amino acid associated with risk of heart disease and strokes and there is evidence that it may also have a role in the prevention of obesity and type 2 diabetes. It is one of the nutrients that is most often absent from diets. The main sources of food folate include dark green leafy vegetables such as spinach and turnip greens, mustard greens, as well as beans, pea and oranges. Cereal grass is also a good source of folate.

Vitamin C

Vitamin C, also known as L-ascorbic acid, is perhaps the best water soluble anti-oxidant in nature. Unlike most animals, humans are unable to synthesize this vitamin, so it is an essential dietary component.

Together with other anti-oxidants, such as vitamin E, β-carotene and selenium, vitamin C reduces free radicals, which damage cells and cellular membranes and contributes to carcinogenesis and the aging process. Vitamin C deficiency causes scurvy, a serious disease in which defective collagen prevents the formation of strong connective tissue. It is essential for the healing of wounds and the formation of scar tissue, as well as for enhancing the body's overall resistance to diseases. Research shows its usefulness in lowering serum uric acid levels, resulting in lower incidence of gout. In addition to its antioxidant and biosynthetic functions, the importance of vitamin C has also been emphasized as it plays an important role in immune function and improves the absorption of non-heme iron, the form of iron present in plant-based foods.

The best sources of vitamin C are fruits and vegetables, among which citrus fruits, kiwi fruit, red and blue berries, red pepper, broccoli, brussels sprouts, cabbage, tomato and cereal grass.

Vitamin E

Vitamin E is a fat-soluble vitamin that includes four tocopherols and four trocotrienols. The α-tocopherol form is the most abundant form in nature, showing a very high biological activity and reversing vitamin E deficiency symptoms in humans.

Vitamin E prevents the spread of free-radical reaction in the human body, by acting as a chain-breaker, thus contributing to prevent several chronic diseases, mainly those believed to have an oxidative stress component, such as cardiovascular diseases, atherosclerosis and cancer. Although vitamin E may be provided from a variety of food sources, α-tocopherol is more abundantly found in nuts, seeds and vegetable oils.

This vitamin is also present in green leafy vegetables, tomato, kiwi fruit and mango, and an analog of α-tocopherol has also been isolated from barley grass.

Vitamin K

Vitamin K, a fat soluble vitamin necessary for the formation of prothrombin, a chemical required in blood clotting which is crucial for the prevention of hemorrhage and excessive blood loss and also required for the synthesis of several important proteins such as osteocalcin, involved in bone metabolism. It has been used for reducing excessive menstrual flow and cramps, and often given to newborn infants to prevent the hemorrhagic disease, sometimes associated with the first weeks of life.

Before this vitamin could be easily synthesized, several medical studies reported the excellent recovery of patients submitted to liver or gallbladder surgery, who were given dehydrated cereal grass (Cerophyl) before surgery. In fact, this supplement was a very rich source of vitamin K and, as described later, completely nontoxic, even in high doses, in opposition to its synthetic forms.

Leafy green vegetables, including collard greens, spinach and green salads, as well as soy and canola oils are rich dietary sources of vitamin K. Cereal grass has also been pointed out as a good source of vitamin K.

Minerals

Minerals are constituents of bones, teeth, soft tissue, muscles, blood and nerve cells, and "green food" contains a great diversity of these micronutrients, such as Calcium Iron, Phosphorus, Potassium, Magnesium, Manganese, Selenium, Sodium Zinc, Copper and Cobalt, their concentration depending on several factors, including growing conditions and growth stage at which they were harvested. Among these minerals, only Calcium and Iron will be highlighted in the following paragraphs.

Calcium

From all minerals in the human body, calcium is the most abundant. In fact, 99% of the body's calcium supply is stored in the bones and teeth, whereas the remaining 1% is required to support several metabolic functions, such as nerve transmission, muscle function, intracellular signaling, hormonal secretion and vascular contraction and vasodilatation. To maintain constant concentrations of calcium in blood, muscle, and intercellular fluids, the human body uses bone tissue as a reservoir and source of calcium. Actually, throughout life, there is a continuous process of reabsorption and deposition of calcium into bone. In periods of growth in children and adolescents, bone formation exceeds reabsorption, whilst a balance in the processes is generally observed in early and middle adulthood. Finally, in aging adults, mainly in postmenopausal women, there is a raise in bone loss, due to bone breakdown exceeding formation, increasing the risk of osteoporosis.

Dairy products are often mentioned as the main source of natural calcium. However, nondairy sources can also contribute with calcium to the diet, and they include vegetables, such as spinach, turnip greens, broccoli, Chinese cabbage, kale, and broccoli. Cereal grass has also been considered a good calcium source, and foods fortified with calcium can also be a supplementary source of this mineral. Different kinds of beans and hulled sesame seeds are other nondairy foods in which calcium is present in large amounts.

Vitamin D improves calcium absorption, while high protein diets are thought to reduce the absorption of this mineral. Plant components, such as phytic and oxalic acids, bind to calcium and can inhibit its absorption. However, the extent to which these compounds affect calcium absorption varies. Some leafy greens such as spinach and collard greens, as well as rhubarb, sweet potato and cocoa have high levels of oxalic acid, while phytic acid can be found in fiber-containing whole-grain products and wheat bran, beans, seeds, nuts, and soy, among others. On the contrary, dehydrated cereal grasses could be considered a good calcium source, as they contain only small amounts of oxalic acid, thus making calcium absorption more efficient.

Despite the fact that calcium from some plant foods is well absorbed, consuming enough plant foods to achieve the Recommended Dietary Allowance (RDA) may be unrealistic for many. Some studies, however, indicate that in African populations, calcium supplied by a number of green leafy plants can be absorbed in quantities comparable to the calcium absorbed from dairy products, and in many areas of the world where dairy products are rarely consumed, osteoporosis is uncommon.

Iron

From all metals on earth, iron is one of the most abundant and essential for the majority of life forms. In humans, besides playing a vital role in regulating cell differentiation and growth, and being an important component of enzymes that support biochemical reactions, its main role is related to oxygen transport to the body tissues, as it is a fundamental constituent of proteins such as hemoglobin and myoglobulin. It is also essential for antibody production, DNA and RNA synthesis, β-carotene conversion into vitamin A and drugs detoxification in the liver.

A lack of iron conditions the oxygen supply to cells, inducing anemia, abnormal fatigue, reduced work capacity and increased susceptibility to infection, as well as a deficiency in major physiological processes in the human body. On the other hand, excess amounts of iron may induce toxicity and even death.

There are two forms of iron in the human diet: the non-heme and the heme form. The first, less readily absorbed, is present in all plant foods, dairy products, eggs meat, poultry and fish, while the latter, derived from hemoglobin and better absorbed, is only naturally present in meat, poultry and fish, in about 50% of their total iron content, the other 50% being non-heme, as mentioned previously.

Among the main iron sources of vegetal origin are soybeans, lentils, spinach rice, maize, black beans, soybeans, wheat and raisins; cereal grasses are also considered a good source of iron.

Chlorophyll

Chlorophyll is the green pigment of plants critical in photosynthesis, a chemical process in which the energy absorbed from light converts carbon dioxide into organic chemical compounds, especially carbohydrates, and oxygen. It is usually found associated with vitamin K in the chloroplasts of green plants and its derivatives are believed to be among the family of phytochemical compounds potentially responsible for associating diets rich in fruits and vegetables with prevention of chronic diseases.

The therapeutic properties of chlorophyll have long been investigated and numerous benefits have been ascribed to this green pigment. One of them derives from the similarity in the chemical structures of chlorophyll and heme, a component of hemoglobin. This fact led some early authors to consider cereal grass and other dark green plants as "blood-building" foods.

Further studies suggest that some porphyrins, the ringed structures in heme and chlorophyll, stimulate the synthesis of the protein portion of the hemoglobin molecule and so, parts of the chlorophyll molecule could stimulate the production of hemoglobin by the human body. This fact might, in part, explain the alleged role of chlorophyll on hemoglobin synthesis. However, despite all the studies performed, the correlation between chlorophyll and heme molecules, is still not completely clear.

Other benefits of chlorophyll such as improving chronic and acute sinusitis, chronic rectal lesions and vaginal infections, speeding the healing of chronic ulcers, anti-bacterial effect and wound healing can also be mentioned.

According to the 2010 "Dietary Guidelines for Americans", there are three main reasons supporting the need to eat more vegetables and fruits:

- Most vegetables and fruits are excellent sources of the most important nutrients, several of which frequently under consumed, such as dietary fiber, several vitamins, such as vitamins A, C, K and folate, and minerals like magnesium and potassium. Some of these nutrients are considered of public concern for the general public by the US Department of Health and Human Services (e.g. dietary fiber), and others for specific groups (e.g. folic acid for women that may become pregnant).

- Consumption of vegetables and fruits has been linked with reduced risk of several chronic diseases. Evidence suggest that the intake of (at least) 2 ½ cups of vegetables and fruits per day reduces the risk of cardiovascular diseases, and may also have a protective action against some types of cancer.

- Vegetables and fruits, raw or prepared, without the addition of fats or sugars, are in general relatively low in calories so their consumption, instead of high caloric foods, will help both children and adults to maintain a healthy weight.

Attention should be drawn to fruit and cereal juices. In fact, although a healthy diet may include them it should be emphasized that using centrifugal / masticating juicers will destroy the majority of the dietary fiber present in these food sources. Fruit juices should be 100% natural, derived from whole fruit and without the addition of sugars.

Still according to the same source, very few Americans consume the amounts of vegetables recommended as part of healthy eating patterns, and a similar situation (occurs in many different parts of the world.

Super Foods

There are foods that exhibit very specific characteristics in terms of boosting the human health and therefore many nutrition experts name them as "Super Foods".

The list below presents some of these Super Foods, highlighting some of the most important benefits they are responsible for.

FOOD TYPE	BENEFITS
- Aloe Vera	Collagen Production
- Blackberries	Massive Antioxidant High in Minerals
- Brazil Nuts	Source of Selenium Antioxidant High in Minerals
- Cacao: Raw Chocolate	Massive Antioxidant Brain Happiness High in Magnesium
- Camu Camu Berry	High Source of Vitamin C
- Coconut Oil (wild)	Hormone Builder Anti parasitical Anti viral

- Dandelion	Liver Cleanser
- Elderberries	Massive Antioxidant
- Grass	Source of Key Minerals Cleansing properties
- Rocket (salad leaves)	Source of Minerals Chlorophyll
- Sea Weeds (including kelp & dulse)	Source of Minerals Chlorophyll
- Spirulina	Source of Protein Chlorophyll
- Stinging Nettles	Source of Silicon Minerals Chlorophyll

Green vegetable juices

It is of the upmost importance to include raw foods in our daily diet - juicing or blending is an excellent way to receive large quantities of these specific foods; it also makes it possible for busy people to add more of the so-called "healing foods" into their diets.

The main benefits of drinking green vegetable juices / blends on a daily basis are listed below:

- Source of uncorrupted protein (Note that protein is easily corrupted by heat)
- Calming effect
- Source of Iron
- Alkalizing effect – balances your body pH
- Easier to consume and digest than whole leaves
- Muscle building
- Cleansing properties
- Massively high in minerals, especially wild greens and grasses
- Supply huge amounts of antioxidants easily

Nutrient depletion

Heat, air, light and drugs are the main factors for the depletion of nutrients in foods. Juices and blends deteriorate quicker because their protective fiber is removed. When juices or blends are prepared, they should be immediately placed in the freezer, if not promptly consumed. They can also be placed in a thermos flask, filled closer to the top so there is little air in the flask - this will keep the juice or blend really cool, out of light and away from air all day long. Alternatively, ice cubes may be inserted inside in the thermos to lower the juice's temperature, and the thermos must be kept it in the fridge until consumption.

A list of the ingredients that can be used to prepare green drinks in the form of juice or blend is presented below, highlighting some of the benefits of each element:

- **Sprouts:** Contain many vitamins, minerals and micronutrients. They are often called a superfood by excellence.

- **Alfalfa Sprouts:** Help to lower cholesterol, shift weight, and are a source of protein and antioxidants.

- **Boldo:** Helps digestion, protects the liver from toxins, has anti-inflammatory and antimicrobial properties and is believed to stimulate the production of bile while acting as a diuretic.

- **Broccoli:** Strong anti-cancer ingredient. Also helps to cleanse and strengthen the blood, to boost the immune system and to improve digestion. Broccoli helps to lower cholesterol and is an important source of vitamins A, B$_2$, B$_5$, B$_6$, B$_9$ (folic acid) and C, and the minerals Calcium, Iron, Phosphorus, Potassium and Magnesium.

- **Cabbage:** Anti-cancer, source of fiber, contributes to weight loss, strengthens blood and immunity; source of vitamin C and Glutamine, an amino acid, which has anti-inflammatory properties.

- **Celery:** Lowers cholesterol, contributes to weight loss and is a good source of fiber and vitamin C. A note must be made to subjects allergic to celery, for whom exposure can cause potentially anaphylactic shock - in the European Union, foods that contain or may contain celery, even in trace amounts, have to be clearly marked as such.

- **Dandelion Greens:** Excellent at warding off cancer, strengthening the immune system and also helping with weight loss and cholesterol levels. They are a good source of luteolin - an antioxidant, and a great source of Iron and Calcium.

- **Kale:** Also an anti-cancer, it lowers cholesterol, strengthens blood and immunity, contributes to weight loss and contains vitamins A, C, K, lutein, and zeaxanthin, as well as Iron, Calcium, Potassium and Magnesium.

Please Note: Because of its high vitamin K content, patients taking anti-coagulants such as warfarin are encouraged to avoid this food since it increases the vitamin K concentration in the blood, which is what the drugs are often attempting to lower.

- **Kelp:** Strengthens the blood and immune system whilst lowering cholesterol and assisting in the breakdown of proteins and the regeneration of blood cells. It is also a source of vitamins B_2, B_5 and B_9 and of the minerals Iron, Calcium, Magnesium and Iodine.

- **Lemon Grass:** Aids in digestion, reduces fevers, flu symptoms, headaches and intestinal irritation. It also has antifungal properties.

- **Oat Grass:** As with watercress, but also contains a high level of fiber, Iron and Magnesium.

- **Okra:** Anti-cancer, strengthens blood and immunity, improves digestion, lowers cholesterol and contributes to weight loss. It is a good source of fiber, vitamins C, B_1, B_6, B_9 and the minerals Iron, Calcium and Magnesium.

- **Papaya:** Aids digestion; eliminates heartburn,

indigestion and inflammatory bowel diseases.

- **Parsley:** Anti-cancer, it strengthens blood and immunity, lowers cholesterol, and contributes to weight loss. It is a good source of vitamins A, B_2, B_9 and C and the minerals Calcium, Iron, Magnesium and Potassium. It has diuretic effects, stimulates digestion and helps kidney, liver, stomach, lung and thyroid functions.

- **Pau d'Arco:** Immune stimulant, effective against bacterial, fungal, viral, parasitic and yeast infections.

- **Peppermint:** Treats colicky pain, irritable bowel syndrome, indigestion, gall stones, candida, yeast infections, and relieves mucus congestion. Other health benefits are attributed to the high content of Manganese and vitamins A and C, as well as trace amounts of various other nutrients such as fiber, Iron, Calcium, Folate, Potassium, Magnesium, Copper, Tryptophan, Omega-3 fatty acids and Riboflavin.

- **Rosehips:** Relaxes stomach, stimulates circulation and digestion, and detoxifies the liver. It also shows antioxidant properties, and fights inflammation, bacteria and fungi.
- **Spinach:** Anti-cancer, improves digestion and

blood pressure, strengthens blood and immunity, lowers cholesterol and contributes to weight loss. It is a good source of fiber, vitamins A, B9, E, and K, several antioxidants and the minerals Calcium, Iron, and Magnesium. On the down side, it contains high levels of Oxalate which binds to iron and calcium, decreasing its absorption, a fact that needs to be taken into consideration when consuming large amounts of this leafy vegetable.

- **Thyme:** Antiseptic, treats respiratory problems such as asthma, allergies and coughs, as well as digestive problems and headaches.

- **Tomato:** Anti-cancer, lowers cholesterol, strengthens blood and immunity, contributes to weight loss, source of vitamins A and C as well as Licopene, a powerful antioxidant, and the minerals Iron and Potassium.

- **Watercress:** Strong cancer fighting capabilities; helps reducing cholesterol and aids with weight reduction. It contains significant amounts of Iron, Calcium and Folic acid, in addition to vitamins A and C.

Vegetables, fruit and antioxidants

Oxidative stress may, in part, account for the development of several chronic and degenerative diseases such as cancer, heart diseases, Parkinson's and Alzeimer's diseases, as well as in the aging process. Several systems in the human body contribute to the elimination of free radicals; they are, however, not totally effective. We can protect against free radicals with antioxidants that may be synthesized in the body or obtained from the foods we eat.

Like the apple that is cut, rubbing on it some lemon juice containing Vitamin C (a water soluble antioxidant), will stop the apple from browning and deteriorating at anywhere near the speed it would do normally without the lemon juice. When we provide a regular intake of antioxidants to our body, the rate at which we age and degenerate decreases dramatically... and so do our chances of getting any form of disease.

Antioxidants are naturally occurring in many fruits, vegetables and herbs. They used to be measured in terms of milligrams of weight of isolated vitamins such as Vitamin C, Vitamin E etc; however, a relatively new research tool designed by G. Cao at the National Institute on Aging in Baltimore, Maryland and further developed by R. Prior and collaborators at Jean Mayer USDA Human Nutrition Research Center on Aging at

Tufts University, Boston, measures the total amount of antioxidant capacity in a food as a whole, rather than individual quantities of isolated antioxidants. The test is known as ORAC, which stands for Oxygen Radical Absorbency Capacity. The higher the ORAC score signifies how well nature endowed that food with overall powers to neutralize cell damaging free radicals. Highest are fruits, vegetables and herbs – the higher in ORAC score the foods you eat, the better.

The table shown in the last chapter: *Useful Resources,* shows the key ORAC values from fruits, vegetables and herbs presented by scientists from the United States Department of Agriculture on the "USDA Database for the Oxygen Radical Absorbance Capacity". Values are expressed as the "total ORAC", which is the sum of the lipid soluble (i.e. carotenoid) and water-soluble (e.g. phenolic) antioxidant fractions, and reported as in micromoles TROLOX equivalents (TE) per 100 gram samples.

On a super-nutritional diet, it is the highly nutritious, low calories and the high antioxidant foods that are of importance.

Sea Vegetables

All of the essential elements for human health are

present in sea vegetables, including Calcium, Magnesium, Potassium, Iodine, Iron, and Zinc, together with important trace elements (such as Selenium), that are often lacking in land vegetables due to soil demineralization.

The minerals in sea vegetables exist in a chelated, colloidal form that makes them readily 'bioavailable' for use in crucial bodily functions. Population studies show that people with a regular intake of sea vegetables show few symptoms of mineral depletion. The longevity of the people of Okinawa is believed to be due to their regular consumption of sea vegetables.

Several decades ago, dietary researcher W. Price found that natives of the high Andes carried a small bag attached to their necks containing a greenish-brown substance, a quantity of which was consumed every day. This substance was sea vegetable obtained with much difficulty from coastal areas, but which these healthy dwellers of the high Andes would not do without.

Low mineral foods are a result of decades of over farming soils. Instead, farmers just add nitrogen and potassium to make the plants look good. This practice leads to woefully inadequate levels of minerals being present in our foods. Since the sea contains an abundant supply of all 92 minerals, plants that grow in the sea are natural sources minerals.

Sea vegetables add a very salty element to any recipe, so make sure to use them sparingly as a condiment, or balance the strong salt taste out with sweet flavors such as carrots and red bell peppers.

FOOD-BIOAVAILABILITY & WATER

In pharmacology, bioavailability is used to describe the fraction of an administered dose of unchanged drug that reaches the systemic circulation. Bioavailability of a nutrient on the other hand, is a measure of the efficiency of delivery (absorption) of that nutrient; how much of what is ingested is actually used by the body. The remaining amount is removed as waste as it cannot be metabolized.

Several factors may affect the bioavailability of a nutrient, such as a physiologic condition (e.g. aging, pregnancy), a disease state or even gender. The presence of some substances may also influence bioavailability. In fact, when taken with fatty foods, calcium and magnesium loose part of their effectiveness. Nevertheless, eating foods in liquid format allow us to absorb their nutrients and minerals in a faster and more efficient way by removing the need for the stomach to break up the fiber, resulting in an increase of the bioavailability of amino acids, minerals and all other nutrients contained in the food.

Water

According to the water specialists, drinking an adequate amount of water each day assists the body to maintain good health.

The human body is two-thirds water; water is essential and is involved in every function of the body. It helps transport nutrients and waste products in and out of cells; it is necessary for all digestive, absorption, circulatory and excretory functions, as well as for the utilization of water-soluble vitamins. It is also needed for the maintenance of proper body temperature, a very sensitive issue for the human body.

Nutritionists have difficulty in suggesting an exact daily requirement because the amount of water needed varies, depending on the climate and whether any type of activity is undertaken. Even on cool days and shorter workouts, one may still need to drink more than non-athletes. The best way to get this water is by drinking plain water. Other beverages, such as "real" fruit and vegetable juices are also good sources of water. Alcoholic beverages, whilst supplying water to the body initially, they often contain diuretics that cause the body to lose water faster than it should.

We can go without food for a month or longer, but we cannot do without water for more than two to five days. Dehydration symptoms generally become noticeable after around two per cent of one's normal water volume has been lost. Initially, one experiences thirst and discomfort, possibly along with loss of appetite and dry skin. Symptoms of dehydration may include headaches, sudden experiences of visual snow, lower blood pressure and a sensation of dizziness or feelings similar to fainting. Symptoms of mild dehydration include thirst, decreased urine volume, tiredness and irritability, severe headaches, dry mouth, and, in some cases, the experience of sleeping disorders. Other symptoms of dehydration may include lethargy and extreme sleepiness.

Symptoms become increasingly severe with greater water loss. One's heart and respiration rates begin to increase to compensate for decreased plasma volume and blood pressure, while body temperature may rise due to decreased sweating. With ten to fifteen per cent fluid loss, muscles may become spastic, vision may dim, urination may be greatly reduced and one may experience delirium sensations. Losses greater than thirteen to fifteen per cent are usually fatal.

A special caution note is to be given regarding this topic to people aged 50+. The body's thirst sensation diminishes with age, hence the reason for having many senior citizens suffering from symptoms of dehydration without knowing. Adding alcohol to this equation may be fatal.

A straightforward plan to keep hydrated:

- Drink at least 1.5lt of water each day. The more the activity the more water is needed to replenish lost fluids.

- Start and end any day with water. The body looses water whilst sleeping hence the importance of drinking water (even if just half glass) prior to bedtime and immediately after waking up.

- Don't wait for the feeling of thirst. By the time one feels thirsty one has probably lost two or more cups of total body water composition.

- When exercising, drink water throughout the workout. Keep a bottle of water close by and take frequent water breaks.

- Don't underestimate the amount of fluids lost from perspiration. Following a workout, drink plenty of water until thirst has been quenched.

- Common colds and the flu frequently lead to dehydration. Keep a large bottle of water next to the bed to sip it throughout the day

- Make sure children drink enough water. Children need water to balance their intake of other beverages – especially during activities.

It is almost impossible to drink too much water, although if large volumes of water are taken in a short space of time it can provide short lived symptoms similar to being drunk.

A QUICK WORD ON DIETS

Note: any food plan, either permanent or temporary, is technically called a "diet", hence the terms *ketogenic diet, Mediterranean diet, vegetarian diet, Okinawa diet...*

It is hard to find any area where half as much contradictory advice is available as when comes to food. With such a profusion of information, we must too often expect to find ignorance, mysticism or even secular-based theories, rather than true knowledge.

Many popular diets in circulation recommend eating adequate protein & fat and a low carbohydrate menu and, by this simple formula, live healthily and lose weight. This so-called ketogenic diet (its medical name) was developed in the early 1920s and may be useful, in specific occasions and when properly handled.

A common problem with this diet lies in the fact that it may induce serious dehydration. While strictly following the plan, the dieter's weight will go down, as witnessed by the scale . However, when the dieter goes back on a balanced schedule of eating, the cells of the body will again able to hold the water they want, and the scales will go bouncing back up, much to the dieter's regret.

Vegetarianism

George Bernard Shaw, Mahatma Gandhi and Bernard MacFadden would all be called food faddists by many health experts. We know that they all reached old age in excellent health, with at least as much mental alertness at 75 as exhibited in their early years. It would not be wise, in a study on longevity, to ignore their diets and thoughts on food; they all made crusades of their eating habits and attempted to get others to join them.

These men were, for most of their lives, vegetarians. Gandhi ate meat for a few years, but could never force himself to like the taste of it. The other two never touched meat during their adult life. Mahatma Gandhi was undoubtedly the most famous person to fast in our times - He had fasted many times before beginning to make political capital out of his refusal to eat. His mother had quite often fasted during his boyhood for religious reasons.

Within this equation, a note should be expressed: there is nothing medically wrong with such a vegetarian diet. Advice on specific diets should be devised to cater for specific lifestyles. Many people enjoy the taste of meat and fish whilst others prefer the vegetarian, the vegan and the raw cuisine. Our bodies are wonderful mechanisms and they can digest and manufacture nearly all the correct chemicals we need for good nutrition. They need only be given the proper nutrients from which to derive energy and cell replacement elements.

The Okinawa diet

The Okinawa diet is a nutrient-rich and low-calorie diet from the indigenous people of the Ryukyu Islands. The traditional diet of the islanders was twenty per cent lower in calories than the Japanese average and contained approximately three hundred per cent of the green & yellow vegetables of that of their fellow countrymen. While the traditional Japanese diet included large quantities of rice, in Okinawa rice was consumed in smaller amounts and the staple was instead the sweet potato. This diet has approximately twenty five per cent of the sugar and around seventy five per cent of the grains in comparison to the average Japanese dietary intake. The traditional diet also included a relatively small amount of fish (less than half a serving per day) and a considerable amount of legumes. Animal protein, such as fish, was primarily eaten on holidays and the everyday diet was almost exclusively plant based.

In addition to their high life expectancy, islanders are known for their low mortality from cardiovascular disease and certain types of cancers. The main principle of this diet divides food into four categories based on caloric density. The "featherweight" foods, less than or equal to 0.8 calories per gram which one can eat freely without major concern, the "lightweight" foods with a caloric density from 0.8 to 1.5 calories per gram which one should eat in moderation, the "middleweight" foods with a caloric density from 1.5 to 3.0 calories per gram which one should eat only while carefully monitoring portion size and the "heavyweight" foods from 3 to 9 calories per gram which one should eat only occasionally.

The Mediterranean diet

On November 17, 2010, UNESCO recognized this diet as an Intangible Cultural Heritage of Italy, Greece, Spain and Morocco, reinforcing it as a great contribution to the world. The most commonly understood version of this diet was presented, by Dr Walter Willett of Harvard University's School of Public Health. Based on "food patterns typical of Crete, Greece, and southern Italy in the early 1960s", this diet, in addition to "regular physical activity," emphasizes "abundant plant foods, fresh fruit as dessert, olive oil as the principal source of fat, dairy products (principally cheese and yogurt), fish and poultry consumed in low to moderate amounts, zero to four eggs consumed weekly, red meat consumed in low amounts, and wine consumed in low to moderate amounts".

The principal aspects of this diet include high olive oil consumption, high consumption of legumes, high consumption of unrefined cereals, high consumption of fruits, high consumption of vegetables, moderate consumption of dairy products (mostly as cheese and yogurt), moderate to high consumption of fish, low consumption of meat and meat products, and moderate wine consumption.

Fasting as a temporary diet

Occasional fasting as a way of life, as well as a temporary diet and a way of weight control is an old concept. Today it is being sold as a great revelation in many healthy-related publications.

Fasting was not invented in 1963, or in any other period of history. The situation – consuming no food - is no different from being really poor. In many parts of the world, for example, periods of starvation are still common. The long-lived Hunzingas are a true example of this. In the autumn, food runs out. For some there may be a sustenance level of food left, but for many there is none. Yet, these people are famous for virility and activity beyond their nineties and hundreds. Obviously this problem of three square meals a day is not solved in their mode of life - but their length of life looks far better than it does for many of the so-called "well fed." All in all, there is nothing mysterious or occult about fasting. Most people in good health can undertake a brief one to three day fast period with safety. Please note that one should not proceed with any fasting-related program without consulting a physician.

The so-called "crash diets"

Crash diets (of which fasting is the most dramatic) are usually neither a permanent nor a satisfactory way to lose weight. The choice for a specific food and relying solely on it for a period of time may prove unwise and even dangerous in certain conditions. Habits are not changed in days, and the unexpressed hope of the crash diet is always that habits will be changed without effort. This is simply a case in which another form of wishful thinking is substituted for hard, cold logic.

The role of the glands

"It's my glands" is a favorite complaint of many; in very few cases this statement may be true, and the more over-weight the person is - say, forty, fifty, sixty pounds overweight - the more likely this is to be true. However, even in these circumstances, overeating may have caused the very failure of these glands that lead to a never-ceasing spiral of more and more weight. Glands can only operate best when we are of normal/adequate size for our body structure. The bigger we get, the harder these glands must work and so, increasing one's weight equates to a more active part of our glands, many times burdened beyond their capacity.

Diabetes – a condition that has been skyrocketing world wide - is more commonly found in the obese. One type of this diabetic condition is caused by a gland failure. The pancreas, the organ that manufactures insulin, becomes exhausted by being too long overtaxed, and simply quits working.

Apparently this same problem of exhaustion can happen with other glands like the thyroid, one of the largest endocrine glands. In most cases, excess weight is simply caused by over eating and can be corrected by the commitment to a basic exercise & nutrition plan.

Hereditary and weight

There are families of overweight people, but this does not mean that this condition runs in the family. What it does mean is that in such a group, eating, as an end to itself, may be being used as a substitute expression of love, reward, and attention…it may also be the case that some people love their food – too much!

PART V

FINAL NOTES: THE STARTING POINT
AUTHOR'S FINAL REMARKS
WORLD HEALTH ORGANIZATION STRATEGY

AUTHOR'S FINAL REMARKS

Health status is significantly influenced by food choices and physical activity. Food plays a direct role in nutritional health, and it is very important that each one takes personal responsibility for his own health. However, the individual capacity to choose what to eat, and the availability of the different kinds of foods are influenced by economic and social factors, together with physical environment conditions. These environmental and social changes that influence eating patterns and physical activity have had a paramount influence on the increasing values regarding overweight and obesity.

Nutrition & food

A super-nutritional diet is highly nutritious, low in calories and high in antioxidant foods. Whole grains, fresh fruits and vegetables all add up to skin cleansing and contribute to optimum health. Strive to eat foods as close to their natural state as possible, but start with easily digestible foods such as spinach and salads.

- Green vegetables: aside from maintaining body weight at low levels, green vegetables also help to release toxins and provide the required daily nutrients, enzymes, vitamins and minerals.

- Omega fatty acids: found in flax seeds, walnuts, almonds, salmon, deep ocean fish, avocadoes, and other rich sources. They are pivotal for healthy skin and for the brain. They also help the skin fight the free radical damage.

- Antioxidant rich foods: blueberries, raspberries, blackberries, cranberries, goji berries, açai berries and spices such as cinnamon and turmeric are an excellent option to fight free radicals. Antioxidants can also be found in broccoli, spinach, tomatoes, and garlic. They literally cleanse the body of toxins and other by-products of cell metabolism that can cause aging. They also contain high levels of rich nutrients, vitamins, and minerals that feed and nourish the skin.

- Avocado: Abundant source of vitamin E which is indispensable for lustrous skin and shiny hair. It also helps to keep those wrinkles off the face.

- Ginger: Facilitates digestion and keeps bowel movement in shape, thereby enabling good gut health.

- Nuts & seeds: eating nuts regularly will help fighting lethargy and packs the body with optimum energy.

- Adequate amount of protein: eat a good amount of protein; if you do not eat animal protein, it is important to learn how to include the essential amino-acids in your daily diet.

Exercise

Exercise produces a flush and makes us sweat. It helps to keep the skin clean and nourished so that it looks younger and more vibrant. Aim for at least 30 minutes of exercise three to five times per week. Remember to also include an appropriate weight-training exercise routine to burn fat faster and to assist in sculpting the body. Exercise regularly, incorporating stretching, aerobics, and strength training.

Personal psychology

This is probably the key to keep healthy and looking wonderful both inside and outside. This is what keeps us on track and what helps us to progressively making changes to healthier lifestyles and to derive the same, if not more pleasure out of it. Latest trends in medical research show that mind and body should be treated as a whole.

Water

Drink a good amount of water and water-rich foods (vegetables, fruits...) and keep yourself hydrated at all times. Dehydration causes the body to start shutting down and deteriorating. This means the organs become less able to detoxify the body and dehydrated skin will start looking old and wrinkled. Drink at least one to two litters of water per day.

Fresh air

Have plenty of fresh air, especially if you live in a polluted metropolis like London, New York or Hong Kong. Oxygen enables the cells of the body to release the energy stored as high-energy chemical bonds in our food and enables them to use that energy to do what cells do, namely, to keep us alive, heart beating, brain thinking, etc. Virtually every cell in the body needs oxygen in order to perform its part in the complex symphony that is our human body.

Relax and recover

Learn easy ways to release and to control stress and anxiety to minimize the impact stress has on the body. This can be done with hypnosis, meditation, yoga or other techniques that promote relaxation and some form of mind-body balance.

Massage

Indulge yourself in an ongoing program of massages. In countries where plastic surgery is a must-have procedure, first-class Plastic Surgeons recommend follow-up massage programs to progressively manipulate the tissues. I usually recommend specialized Body-Sculpting massages to enhance aesthetic results.

Facial aerobics

Facial exercises can smooth away the years. Done daily, it can tone muscles underneath the skin. By strengthening these facial muscles you will increase the tonus of the eyes, cheeks, forehead, jaw, and neck. The beauty of face exercises is that they require no expensive health hubs, no top branded creams and no invasive procedures.

Detoxify

The colon, liver, and kidneys have a habit of collecting junk from one's environment and from consumed foods. To learn how to detoxify one's body regularly helps to minimize the feelings of weakness and sluggishness, together with supporting the skin to look younger and more vibrant.

WORLD HEALTH ORGANIZATION GLOBAL STRATEGY ON DIET, PHYSICAL ACTIVITY AND HEALTH

The utmost importance of including more "green food" and fruits in human diet and increasing physical activity is generally recognized, but frequently not implemented. In May 2004, the World Health Assembly adopted the World Health Organization Global Strategy on Diet, Physical Activity and Health, with four main objectives:

- Reduce risk factors for chronic diseases that stem from unhealthy diets and physical inactivity through public health actions.

- Increase awareness and understanding of the influences of diet and physical activity on health and the positive impact of preventive interventions.

- Develop, strengthen and implement global, regional, national policies and action plans to improve diets and increase physical activity that are sustainable, comprehensive and actively engage all sectors.

- Monitor science and promote research on diet and physical activity.

As for the diet, recommendations for populations and individuals should include:

- Achieve energy balance and a healthy weight.

- Limit energy intake from total fats and shift fat consumption away from saturated fats to unsaturated fats and towards the elimination of trans-fatty acids.

- Increase consumption of fruits, vegetables and legumes, whole grains and nuts.

- Limit the intake of free sugars.

- Limit salt (sodium) consumption from all sources and ensure that salt is iodized.

PART VI

USEFUL RESOURCES
RELAXATION TOOLS
EXERCISE PRINCIPLES AND ROUTINES
HEALTHY RECIPES
ORAC TABLE
KITCHEN AIDS

RELAXATION TOOLS

There are plenty of available machines and websites that claim to sell all-purpose products to enhance brain capacity and achieve a pleasant relaxation state - also called homeostasis or the "neutral state". The recommendations below are the result of trial-and-error tests with different devices, websites and products. Many of them were satisfactory, others a complete waste of money & time. Nevertheless, a limited selection passed our test and is our recommendation in this area.

Due to the purpose of this book, the following items are briefly explained to provide an overall note and a short introduction to the below mentioned selection. To keep the reader up-to-date with the latest offers, we have solely included the type of product/website recommended and invite interested parties to visit the website www.thestarbody.com for more detailed information about these types of products, their characteristics and places of sale.

Relaxation can be attained by any method, process, procedure or activity that helps a person to relax and to achieve a state of increased calmness, reducing overall levels of anxiety, stress and anger. Relaxation has been mentioned by different experts as a direct influence in restoring overall psychological health, including increased calm & happiness, clarity, purpose, balance, optimism & energy as well as reduced stress, anxiety, tension, irritability, restlessness & fatigue. Physical benefits include reduced blood pressure and an enhanced immune system.

Since the 1960s, research has indicated strong correlations between chronic stress and physical as well as emotional health. Meditation was amongst the first relaxation techniques shown to have a measurable effect on stress reduction. In the 1970s, self-help books teaching relaxation techniques began to appear on bestsellers lists. In 1975, *The Relaxation Response* by Harvard Medical School professor Herbert Benson, MD and Miriam Z. Klipper was a reference bestseller. Research released in the 1980s indicated stronger ties between stress and health and showed benefits from a wider range of relaxation techniques than had been previously known. This research received national media attention, including a New York Times article in 1986.

Conventional medical philosophy adopted the concept and its early 21st century practitioners recommend using relaxation techniques to improve patient outcomes in many situations. The devices mentioned in this section are for home and personal perusal. Many of them are used by business executives on their ongoing globetrotting travelling schedules.

Recommended relaxation products

Mind relaxation (downloadable audio series)
A blend of proven meditation techniques with stories, music and natural sound effects. Once in a meditative state, one experiences lucid dreaming whilst being in total control. One has the opportunity to create a world within one's imagination. In the suggested programs, content is secular; It is not aligned with any religious, atheist or spiritual movement. These products are often used for personal development and exploration of the mind. Users do this on their own terms.

Head & eye massage helmet
This is one of our favorites. It has received raving reviews and once we tested it, we did not want to give it away. Regular eye massage for 5 to 10 minutes is a good practice to prevent vision problems and help to reduce stress and promote better sleep. It is best for people who use computer monitors for extended periods of time

and for those who suffer from pouchy eyes, dark eye circles, or eye wrinkles caused by tiredness and unsmooth blood circulation. This product is also recommended for people suffering from insomnia, headache, migraines, and presbyopia. The device fully massages the eyes and temples together with head and scalp.

Foot & calf massage
Foot and Calf Massagers offer stimulating roller foot massage, bringing energy and well-being back to tired feet, ankles and legs. Massage technology soothes tired muscles, releases tension and helps improve blood circulation. Foot rollers target vital reflex points on the soles, replicating the push and release technique used by professional reflexologists. Note that any individual who may be pregnant, has a pacemaker and/or suffers from diabetes, phlebitis or thrombosis, is at an increased risk of developing blood clots. Those who have pins/screws/artificial joints or other medical devices implanted in his/her body should consult with a physician before using a massaging device designed for home / personal use.

If we are to exercise correctly, we must understand what the fundamental principles of all exercises are. Once these principles are clear, each of us can evaluate the value of any specific exercise, or of any exercise program.

Strength, agility and endurance are the three principal goals we may wish to derive from exercise. Since no exercise can be done well without strength, much study has been devoted to strength's attainment. During the time of the Greek Olympics, the "training table" was invented; at such a table, the wrestlers were fed a special diet, and its benefits were manifested when these specially-fed athletes won most of their contests. The reasons for this special feeding, and its results, were quite simple. In those golden days there were no weight classifications, and in wrestling the heavier opponent always had an advantage. Once we know the reason for the training table - weight alone - it loses much of its magic.

Strength

Scientific studies beginning after World War II showed that weight lifting, or progressive resistance exercises, were a superior method of gaining strength. There are dozens of books and booklets available on specific weight lifting exercises for each major sport and activity. If weight lifting is to be done satisfactorily and safely, a trainer or coach should set the requirements of each day's effort. Most weight lifters do not undertake any other exercises, but build only strength... and strength alone is only one of the three goals of exercise.

The most effective exercise for strength has been found in *the isometric technique.* In this form of exercise, one simply uses one's own muscles against each other for a single, brief, maximum effort. Research has shown that this isometric technique yields two great advantages: the greatest increase in strength occurs when the single maximum muscular effort is met and sustained up to no more than 6 to 10 seconds. Similar research has shown that an effort of six seconds per exercise may suffice. This increase builds up the fastest when this form of exercise is used only on alternate days.

Isometric exercises are so effective that before the recent Olympics their discovery was "blacked out", censored as too valuable to be released by the Western nations. Isometric exercises are truly a revolution in quick, easy strength-building.

Agility

There are many kinds of exercise for agility. But agility, in itself, is not the average reader's concern; it is mainly the aim of the Olympic and professional athlete.

Agility is simply a speedy, swift muscular response - anatomically applied for a particular athletic situation. This is a desirable attainment for all; it takes a great deal of time and effort to train our bodies and minds to work together to this degree of harmony.

Endurance

Endurance training - the great goal of all fitness for longevity programs - is accomplished by a method exactly the reverse of strength training. Purposeful walking, jogging and running stand very high on the list of good endurance training measures.

Dangerous exercises

Deep knee bends are foremost on the list of those exercises that should be avoided. The knee is the most easily damaged joint in our bodies, and the hardest to heal. A half, or modified knee bend will place all the work on the leg muscles that is needed to give them either strength or endurance. More bending only adds a dangerous load on the knee joint - far more than it was built to endure.

When we engage in a forceful activity - and at the same time stop regular breathing - we also stop the flow of blood into the right side of the heart. The older we are, the more this is apt to cause a heart attack.

Too many of the exercises in vogue today are aimed only at the development of the extremities. Instead, by concentrating on running and walking, jump with a rope and isometric exercises.

"We live in our torso", yet too few exercises are designed to increase the strength of its muscles. Muscles and other tissues will firm up and improve in appearance, but they won't bulge. For many, this new firmness will bring some slight added weight but no added fat at all. This regained attractive appearance applies as much to women as to men.

There has also been a great deal of magical thinking associated with the idea of exercising at some particular time of day. It always seems best to do anything - exercise included - when you feel like it, and to avoid the same activity when you don't; the time of day one does exercise has little scientific evidence on the end results. Incidentally, experience has demonstrated that all exercises are most useful when done to rhythm. You may also prefer to put on your headphones when exercising.

Precautions that should be observed are signs indicating that exercising has been too strenuous:

- Your heart refuses to stop pounding 10 minutes after exercising.

- Your breathing is still uncomfortable 10 minutes after exercising.

- You are still shaky for more than 30 minutes after exercising.

- You cannot sleep well the night after exercising.

- You carry fatigue (not muscle soreness) into the next day.

If any of these symptoms occurs, reduce the number of exercises you do and build up gradually to the former figure over a week or two.

Isometric home-based exercises

- Muscle-strengthening exercise No. 1, for the head and neck muscles: Place your hands with interlocked fingers upon your forehead. The hands should attempt to push the head back out of the way, while the head pushes forward.

- Muscle-strengthening exercise No. 2, for shoulders, Arms and neck: Place your left hand against the left side of your head and push the head onto your right shoulder. Resist this pressure with your neck muscles. Place the right hand against the right side of your head and try to push your head onto your right shoulder. Resist with your neck muscles.

- Muscle strengthening exercise No. 3, to develop the upper chest: Interlock your hands or wrists at chest level with your arms up and your elbows straight out. First push your arms together as vigorously as you are able. Hold this force for six seconds. Then reverse the direction and pull as hard as possible for six seconds.

- Muscle-strengthening exercise No. 4, to develop arms, shoulders, legs, thighs and midsection: While semi-seated, hold the ends of a rope (five to eight feet long depending on your size) firmly in each hand. At the same time, hold the loop of the rope against the soles of your feet. Press against the rope as vigorously as possible with both feet and attempt to pull your feet up with the rope.

- Muscle-strengthening exercises No. 5 & No. 6, for the midsection, abdomen, hips and thighs: Assume a seated position on the floor before a door frame, with your feet resting in the center of the frame. Attempt to push out the door frame with your feet, letting the structure resist. Shift your position to a corner of a wall with one foot on either side of the wall. Squeeze your legs together, letting the structure resist your effort.

- Muscle-strengthening exercise No. 7, to develop legs and shoulders: Stand in a doorway with your hands against the frame and your feet well braced and the right foot forward. Push as hard as you can. Reverse your position so that the left leg takes the position of the right leg, the left arm takes the place of the right. Push again for 6 seconds.

Endurance exercises

Start with 25 minutes a day, 3 to 5 days a week.

- Endurance exercise No. 1, jumping rope: Throw the rope forward and have both your feet leave the ground at the same time. This exercise increases both endurance and agility and since research has shown that exercise done to rhythm is both more enjoyable and useful, the swinging rope will set up a definite rhythm which will promote the physical grace.

- Endurance test No. 2, running: Either running or swimming for 20-plus minutes each exercise day should be your eventual goal. Start by walking briskly and vigorously for ten minutes, then fifteen minutes, then twenty minutes to loosen the muscles and build endurance for running. Once twenty minutes of vigorous walking has been accomplished, trotting should be undertaken. Trot for two, three or four minutes and walk for an equal length of time until a twenty minute period has elapsed. As you progress in your fitness, some of the trotting can be speed up to a good running pace with periods of walking and trotting as before. After a couple of weeks, twenty minutes plus of continuous running should be possible without effort.

Experienced runners mention the advantage of exploring different routes to increase experience enjoyment.

HEALTHY RECIPES

Did you know you can eat chocolate, ice cream, pizza, fruit and vegetable juices, lasagna and at the same time put your health and fitness back on track? Were you aware that just by using healthy ingredients and preparing your food in a healthy way, you supply your body with all the nutrients, vitamins and minerals you need for optimum performance?

This chapter addresses several easy-to-prepare recipes with ingredients one can easily find at any local supermarket.

ENERGY SMOOTHIES
Use a blender to mix the ingredients

BERRY-BOOSTER SMOOTHIE

1/2 cup frozen strawberries
1/2 cup frozen blueberries
1/2 cup frozen raspberries
1/2 cup apple juice
1/2 teaspoon lemon juice
1/2 cup ice

TROPICAL SMOOTHIE

1/4 cup apple juice
1 pinch grated coconut or 1 tablespoon coconut milk
1/2 banana
1/4 teaspoon fresh ginger root peeled
2 ice cubes

TANGO-MORANGO SMOOTHIE

1 banana
1 handful of strawberries
1/2 cup orange juice
A handful of ice cubes

TWISTER SMOOTHIE
1/2 cup orange juice
1 banana
6-7 frozen strawberries
4-5 slices frozen peaches
5-6 frozen blueberries
6-7 ice cubes
Fresh mint (optional)

CHOCOLATE SMOOTHIE
African Raw Chocolate
Almond Milk
1 banana
1 tablespoon Agave Syrup
3 ice cubes

FUZZY-BANANA SMOOTHIE
2 medium bananas quartered
1 pint orange raw sorbet
1 cup mandarin or tangerine juice

SUPER-BERRY SMOOTHIE
1 cup blackberries
1 cup stemmed and halved strawberries
1 cup blueberries
1 cup almond milk
1/8 teaspoon ground cinnamon

TROPICAL-SPLASH SMOOTHIE

1 small banana, peeled and cut into chunks
2 tablespoons coconut milk
2 tablespoons lime juice
1/4 cup orange juice
1/4 cup pineapple juice
1/2 teaspoon ginger
3 ice cubes

ZINGER SMOOTHIE

1 cucumber, peeled, seeded and chopped
3 tablespoons mint leaves & mint sprigs finely chopped
1 1/2 cups apple juice
1 cup lemon raw sorbet
1 cup ice cubes

MELON-MINT SMOOTHIE

1 cup diced honeydew melon
1 cup diced seedless watermelon
1/2 cup passion fruit or mango juice
1 tablespoon lime juice
2 teaspoons honey
10 fresh mint leaves
3 ice cubes

SUNRISE SMOOTHIE
1 banana, peeled and sliced
1/2 cup of strawberries
1/2 cup of orange juice
A handful of ice cubes

APPLE-PINE SMOOTHIE
1/2 cup orange juice
1/4 cup pineapple juice
1/2 banana
1/4 tablespoon pealed fresh ginger root
1/2 cup crushed ice or 2 ice cubes

ISLAND-BERRY SMOOTHIE
1 frozen banana, peeled
1/2 fresh papaya
10-12 raspberries (fresh or frozen)
1/2 cup water or fruit juice

MANGORANGE SMOOTHIE
1/2 cup orange juice
1/2 cup peeled, pitted and sliced fresh mango
Agave Syrup / honey to taste
1/2 cup ice

Place the juice, fruit & honey in a blender. Blend on high speed for 30 sec. Add ice and blend until smooth.

NUTRITIOUS RECIPES

Warm...and still raw: Does raw food have to be cold food? Food is considered raw, providing it has not been heated above 115 degrees Fahrenheit or 47 degrees Celsius; At this temperature, all the enzymes are still active. Chefs usually heat food above 100º C – but by the time it reaches your table it would probably be lower than 47º C.

Below are some ideas on how to keep all the nutrients whilst having warm meals:

- Blended Soups: heat up in a normal saucepan to finger hot temperature.

- Solid foods and vegetables: flash heat in a conventional oven for 1 minute.

- Pre-heat the plates and bowls.

- Heat your vegetables up in finger hot water.

- Add cayenne and chili peppers to your food.

QUINOA AS A SALAD COMPLEMENT

Quinoa seed is light and easily digested. It is gluten free and has the most complete nutrition and highest protein content of any grain, making it an ideal food for vegetarians.

Quinoa is simple to make, cooks very much like rice, and is absolutely delicious all by itself. Cooked quinoa is similar to couscous, but more substantial, tasty and nourishing.

Cooking Directions:
1. Soak the quinoa first for 15 min - 1/2 hour in its cooking pot. Soaking loosens up the outer coating of saponin, which can give a bitter taste if not removed.
2. If you don't have time for long soaking, use hot water and soak for five minutes, then give an extra rinse or two.
3. Stir the quinoa with your hand, and carefully pour off the rinsing water, using a sieve at the last.
4. Put the quinoa back in the pot, add more water, and rinse again two or three more times, until the rinse water is pretty clear.
5. Drain quinoa well in the sieve.
6. Place quinoa in the pot, add the water and salt - 1 cup quinoa, 1 1/2 cups cold water and 1/2 teaspoon of salt.

7. Bring to a boil, cover with a tight fitting lid, and turn the heat down to simmer.
8. Cook for 20 minutes.
9. Remove from heat. Allow to sit 5 minutes-lid on.

MIXED SALAD
Wild Garlic – roots, stems, bulbs, sliced
Wild dandelion leaves, chopped
1 cucumber
Red / yellow pepper – diced
Tomatoes – sliced
Black olives
Olive oil and lemon juice to taste

ASIAN SALAD
1 white cabbage – finely sliced
Handful coriander leaves
Cup of finely chopped cucumber
Cup of finely diced tomato
Handful of cashews
1 green chili – finely sliced
Olive oil and lemon juice to taste

NOODLE SALAD
2 cups butternut squash noodles (use noodle machine or grate the squash in a food processor)
1 red pepper, ginger and lemon rind zest

Tamari / Soy sauce
3 spring onions, chopped fine
2 delicatessen coconut
Sesame oil

KALE SALAD
1 bag of kale
1 cup of chopped tomatoes
1 large avocado
Juice of half a lemon
Good sprinkling of garlic infused virgin olive oil, or
  normal virgin olive oil
Big pinch of cayenne pepper
Big pinch of sea salt

Place all ingredients in a bowl. Squeeze and mix with
your hand to wilt the kale and churn the avocado into a
creamy sauce. Serve immediately.

BROCCOLI AND SATAY SAUCE

Broccoli florets from 2 heads of broccoli

For Satay Sauce
1 inch of ginger
2 tablespoons raw almond butter
1 red chili
1 tablespoon Tamari sauce

3 dates, pitted
1 big garlic clove
Dash of water
Blend all ingredients, add water to make sufficiently
runny and pour it over broccoli

SUNFLOWER PATÉ
2 Cups sunflower seeds and/or pumpkin seeds, soaked
  4 hours
1/3 cup lemon juice
1/4 cup olive oil
1/4 red onion, chopped
2-3 cloves garlic, crushed
Pinch of Rock Salt
1/8 tablespoon cayenne pepper
4-6 Spring onions
¼ cup herbs, chopped (parsley, coriander, oregano,
  basil etc.) and some water

Place the first seven ingredients in a food processor and
process until smooth. Add the spring onions and herbs
and process until well incorporated leaving the herbs a
bit chunky and the paté white (not green). Decorate
with fresh herbs. Serve with flax crackers.

"CANELLONI" APPETIZERS

3 courgettes sliced length ways with a mandolin or potato peeler

For the filling:
2 cups of almonds soaked overnight
1 cup of pine nuts
2 tablespoons of olive oil
2 tablespoons of lemon juice
½ tsp salt
1 or 2 garlic cloves
1/3 teaspoon black pepper
½ teaspoon cayenne pepper
½ cup black olives
1 tablespoon fresh thyme, minced
2 tablespoons fresh basil, minced

Chop up the olives coarsely either by hand or in a food processor. Take out and set aside. Put the soaked almonds and pine nuts through a powerful blender to homogenize the cream. A food processor can also be used. Place the homogenized nut mix in the food processor with everything else apart from the fresh herbs and olives. Mix together well. Mix in the fresh herbs and olives by hand

To Assemble:
Lay down a curgette strip onto a flat surface. Place the filling mixture at one end and roll it up, securing with a

toothpick if necessary. Place in a dehydrator (alternatively use an oven at the lowest possible heat and leave the oven door open) from 1 to 6 hours. Serve warm.

VEGETARIAN MEAT BALLS
1 cup walnuts, soaked overnight
1 cup almonds, soaked overnight
1 cup mushrooms, chopped fine
½ cup grated carrot
1 tablespoon dark miso
¼ minced onion
2 tablespoon Tamari / Soy sauce

Homogenize nuts in a blender (or process fine in food processor). Mix in all other ingredients and dehydrate for a few hours or cook at low heat.

AVOCADO AND CHILI SOUP
2 ripe avocados
3 cups soy milk
1/4 ounce can of green chilies
1/2 onion, chopped
Salt and pepper, to taste
2 tablespoons lime juice
2 tablespoons chopped fresh cilantro

Preparation:
In a food processor or blender, mix together all ingredients except cilantro until smooth. Stir in the cilantro at the end and serve chilled.

TOMATO SAUCE
1 cup of chopped fresh tomatoes
2 cups of sun dried tomatoes. Soak for 3 hours in water
1 tablespoon of date paste
¼ small onion
¼ cup olive oil
1 teaspoon of Himalayan rock salt
½ teaspoon black pepper
Pinch hot pepper flakes
Blend all and serve with meatballs

"TAGLIATELLE" WITH TRUFFLE CREAM SAUCE
Slice 5 courgettes on mandolin with Tagliatelle setting. If desired use a peeler to get the green skin off the courgette first.

Sauce:
1/2 cup cashews
1 teaspoon truffle infused olive oil
1 teaspoon nutritional yeast
1/2 cup water
1/4 teaspoon salt
Blend all and pour over "tagliatelle"

LEAFY GREEN SALAD

Mix together a variety of leafy greens, e.g.

Lambs lettuce

Spinach

Flat lettuce

Rocket

EASY SALAD DRESSING

1½ cups olive oil

½ cup fresh squeezed lemon juice

2 tablespoon finely minced ginger

3 finely minced garlic cloves

HEALTHY SNACKS

Our suggestions for healthy snacks are:

NUTS AND SEEDS (eat them individually / mix)
- Pumpkin seeds
- Sunflower seeds
- Sesame seeds (shelled)
- Brazil nuts
- Almonds
- Hazelnuts
- Cache Nuts

CHOPPED VEGETABLES
- Cucumber
- Carrots
- Broccoli
- Cauliflower
- Tomato

Be creative and eat your chopped vegetables with a healthy sauce/paste (e.g. humus or sunflower paté).

SMOOTHIES
Use any of the smoothies recipes mentioned in this book or create your own recipes. Be creative: blend a combination of fresh fruits, vegetables, ice cubes and

any other healthy ingredient to create highly nutritional smoothies,

FRESH PRESSED FRUIT & VEGGIE JUICES
Use either a masticating or a centrifugal juicer. The goal is to nourish your body with ready-to-absorb, fresh and raw nutrients that will skyrocket your health.

MINT-CHOCOLATE ICE CREAM
4 frozen yellow bananas (ripe)
Handful of fresh mint
1 bottle of Agave syrup
1/3 cup of raw cacao nibs
1 tablespoon coconut oil

Chop the mint finely into a container – you may opt for putting a sweetener such as date paste or honey. Leave it in the fridge for one day to infuse the sweetener with the mint flavor. Mix frozen bananas, coconut oil, 4 tablespoons of the mint infused sweetener and 2 table spoons of the chopped mint from the mint syrup jar.

Blend in a powerful blender or in a food processor. Add in the cacao nibs mix all the ingredients together until its ready to serve.

BANANA SORBET
6 (or more) frozen bananas
1 tablespoon date paste / honey / grape juice as
  sweetener

Preparation:
This recipe is slightly easier if you peel the bananas before freezing them. Simply gently push the frozen

bananas through a powerful blender or food processor.

RAW CAKE BASE
- Nuts and seeds
- 1 tablespoon date paste
- Soaked flax seeds or coconut oil (for consistency)

Preparation:
Mix all in a food processor. Create biscuits or a base for a cake. Put it in the freezer for cold desert (fill with fruit mousse) or leave it in the oven until crispy and ready to eat.

FRUIT MOUSSE
- Any fruit
- Bananas and / or avocados (for consistency)
- 1 tablespoon date paste or honey

Put it in the freezer and before serving, use a powerful blender, a food processor or a masticating juicer to homogenize.

OXIGEN RADICAL ABSOBANCE CAPACITY (ORAC)
OF SOME FRUITS, VEGETABLES AND HERBS
(Total ORAC Values in μmol TE/100g Sample*)

FRUITS		VEGETABLES & HERBS	
Cranberries (raw)	9090	Ginger (root, raw)	14840
Plums (raw)	6100	Marjoram (fresh)	27297
Blackberries (raw)	5905	Peppermint (fresh)	13978
Raspberries (raw)	5065	Oregano (fresh)	13970

Blueberries (raw)	4669	Garlic (raw)	5708
Pomegranates (raw)	4479	Coriander (leaves, raw)	5141
Strawberries (raw)	4302	Cabbage (red, raw)	2496
Cherries (sweet raw)	3747	Lettuce (red leaf raw)	2426
Raisins (seedless)	3406	Chives (raw)	2094
Goji berry (raw)t	3290	Cauliflower (purple, raw)	2084
Mangosteen (raw)	2510	Beet (raw)	1776

Pears (green cultivars with peel, raw)	2201	Radish (raw)	1750
Oranges (raw)	2103	Lettuce (green leaf raw)	1532
Peaches (raw)	1922	Onion (red)	1521
Grapes (red)	1837	Spinach (raw)	1513
Tangerines (raw)	1627	Alfalfa (sprouts, raw)	1510
Grapefruit (raw)	1548	Broccoli (raw)	1510
Lemons (raw without peel)	1346	Parsley (raw)	1301

*Values presented were obtained from the "USDA Database for the Oxygen Radical Absorbance Capacity" (USDA/ARS, 2010).

Some ORAC charts also include the dried versions of the foods listed here. Drying out of any food will increase its antioxidant score by weight, but the increased score is in relation to the amount of calories it contains.

KITCHEN AIDS

From simple juices to complex tarts and cakes, the use of specific kitchen aids are key for those that wish to get the most out of food.

Juicer

Juicing helps to absorb all the nutrients from vegetables as most of us have impaired digestion as a result of making less-than-optimal food choices over many years. These choices limit the body's ability to absorb all the nutrients from fruit and vegetables. Juicing also enables an increased consumption of optimal amount of vegetables in an efficient manner - experts recommend eating one pound of raw vegetables per 50 pounds of body weight per day and this can be easily accomplished with a quick glass of vegetable juice. Juicing also allows the consumption of a wider variety of vegetables in one's diet: many people eat the same vegetable salads every day and this violates the principle of regular food rotation and increases the chances of developing an allergy to a certain food.

We recommend high-end stainless steel juicers with durable design, stainless steel super fine filters and dishwasher safe parts. These machines are ideal for all natural juices, soups, baby food, sauces and more, without unhealthy preservatives. Providing different centrifugal speed settings allow these products to be extremely versatile juice extractors. The lower speed is for softer fruits and leafy green vegetables whilst the higher speed maximizes extraction from dense foods such as apples and carrots. For the more sophisticated users, a masticating-type machine in addition to a centrifugal unit is also recommended.

Power blender

Research shows that phytonutrients and antioxidants in whole foods can significantly reduce damage to the cells by free radicals. The hard part is getting these essential chemicals into a digestible form as they're locked inside skin, pulp and seeds. Powerful blenders can rupture the cell walls of whole foods to deliver the full benefit of nutrients. A whole food diet rich in fruits, vegetables and whole grains is one of the key pillars to a long and healthy life.

Our recommended blender product lines, the so-called "Power-Blenders" are the ideal equipment for "green smoothies". Just drop anything into this blender and it purees the set into a smoothie consistency. It is the ideal way to increase consumption of fruit and vegetables. Usually a pricey piece of equipment but a definitely "must buy".

Hand blender

Equipped with at least 700-watt motors, hand blenders quickly puree soups, mix beverages, nuts & seeds and more. These blenders usually include powerful choppers for chopping or mincing a wide variety of foods, plus a whisk attachment that allows for optimal whipping results. These units are the ideal portable aids for sauces, cakes and biscuits such as almonds and flax seed delicatessens – made with the aid of a dehydrator.

Sprouter

A seed has many nutritional advantages, but many of them are locked up tight by anti-nutrients (such as phytic acid). Once the germinating process starts, that dormant seed becomes a live plant. By sprouting grains, legumes or seeds, we neutralize not only phytic acid very effectively but also enzyme inhibitors. Seeds, grains and legumes will be much easier to digest after sprouted.

Soaking also assists to diminish some of the fat content of grains and seeds and helps converting dense vegetable protein to simpler amino acids for easier digestion. The more complex carbohydrates in the foods also start to break down into the simpler glucose molecules which in turn will ease their digestion. Chinese used to carry mung beans when on long journeys at sea to sprout and eat as they contained sufficient amount of vitamin C to prevent scurvy.

There are different sprouting units available on the market. Our recommendation is for the electric automatic units with programmable irrigation timers and for hemp bags for small-radicule sprouting seeds such as alfalfa and mung beans. Do include Hydroxide Peroxide on sprouters to minimize mold and other bacteria.

Dehydrator

A food dehydrator is an electrical appliance made for drying food indoors. A dehydrator has an electric element for heat with a fan and vents for air circulation. Dehydrators should be efficiently designed to dry foods quickly; drying removes the moisture from the food so bacteria, yeast and mold cannot grow and spoil the food. Drying also slows down the action of enzymes (naturally occurring substances which cause foods to ripen), but does not inactivate them.
In drying, warm temperatures cause the moisture to

evaporate. Low humidity allows moisture to move quickly from the food to the air. Air current speeds up drying by moving the surrounding moist air away from the food. As drying removes moisture, food becomes smaller and lighter in weight.

9-Tray Food Dehydrators are ideal for families that enjoy healthy eating. These units allow drying any food evenly and efficiently, such as fruits, sprouts, nuts & seeds and vegetables. Dehydrating is a great way to add a new way of consuming foods without damaging valuable nutrients that may be lost during high heat cooking. Dried foods are excellent treats because they hold almost all of their nutritional value and flavor.

These units come with a recipe book that provide all the necessary guidance to produce award-winning recipes.

The End

BIBLIOGRAPHY

BIBLIOGRAPHY

Adzersen K.H., Jess P., Freivogel K.W., Gerhard I. and Bastert G. 2003. Raw and cooked vegetables, fruits, selected micronutrients, and breast cancer risk: a case-control study in Germany. *Nutr. Cancer* **46**(2):131–137.

AMA/CFN (Council on Foods and Nutrition) 1962. The regulation of dietary fat. *Journal of the American Medical Association* **181**: 411-429.

Anderson J. 1986. Fiber and health: an overview. *American Journal of Gastroenterology* **10**:892-897.

Anderson J.W., Baird P., Davis Jr. R.H., Ferreri S., Mary Knudtson M., Koraym A., Waters V. and Williams L.C. 2009. Health benefits of dietary fiber. *Nutrition News* **67**:188-205.

Andrews N.C. 1999. Disorders of iron metabolism. *N. Engl. J. Med.* **341**:1986-1995.

ASPL 2010. Plastic Surgery Procedural Statistics. American Society of Plastic Surgeons. http://www.plasticsurgery.org/News-and-Resources/Statistics.html . Accessed on June 27, 2011.

Barker D., Morris J. and Nelson M. 1986. Vegetable consumption and acute appendicitis in 59 areas in England and Wales. *British Medical Journal of Clinical Research Education* **292**:927-930.

Bar-Sela G., Tsalic M., Fried G. and Goldberg H. 2007. Wheat Grass Juice May Improve Hematological Toxicity Related to Chemotherapy in Breast Cancer Patients: A Pilot Study. *Nutrition and Cancer* **58**(1):43-48.

Beck C. and Scott D. 1974. Enzymes in foods—for better or worse. In: *Food Related Enzymes*. J. Whitaker (Ed.). American Chemical Society. Washington, DC.

Ben-Arye E., Goldin E., Wengrower D., Stamper A., Kohn R. and Berry E. 2002. Wheat grass juice in the treatment of active distal ulcerative colitis: a randomized double-blind placebo-controlled trial. *Scand. J. Gastroenterol.* **37**(4):444-449.

Bendich A. and Shapiro, S. 1986. Effect of beta-carotene and canthaxamin on the immune responses of the rat.

Journal of Nutrition **116**:2254-2262.

Bhaskaram P. 2001. Immunobiology of mild micronutrient deficiencies. *Br. J. Nutr.* **85**:S75-80.

Bing, F. 1939. Accepted Foods - Cerophyll. *The Journal of the American Medical Association* **112**:733.

Bothwell T.H., Charlton R.W., Cook J.D. and Finch C.A. 1979. *Iron Metabolism in Man*. Blackwell Scientific, St. Louis, Oxford.

Buchanan T.W. and Lovallo W.R. 2001. Enhanced memory for emotional material following stress-level cortisol treatment in humans. *Psychoneuroendocrinology* **26**(3):307-317.

Caldwell J. and Jakoby W. (Eds.) 1983. *Biological Basis of Detoxification*. Academic Press. New York.

Calloway D., Newell G., Calhoun W. and Munson A. 1962. Further studies of the influence of diet on radiosensitivity of guinea pigs, with special reference to broccoli and alfalfa. *Journal of Nutrition* **79**:340-348.

Cannon M. and Emerson G. 1939. Dietary requirements of the guinea pig with reference to the need for a special factor. *The Journal of Nutrition* **18**:155-167.

Castelvetro G. 1989. *The Fruits, Herbs and Vegetables of Italy*. Original version 1614, translated by Gillian Riley and published again in 1989, Viking, London.

Cao G., Alessio H. and Cutler R. 1993. Oxygen-radical absorbance capacity assay for antioxidants. *Free Radic. Biol. Med.* **14**(3):303–311.

Chandalia M., Garg A., Lutjohann D., von Bergmann K., Grundy S.M. and Brinkley L.J. 2000. Beneficial effects of high dietary fiber intake in patients with type 2 diabetes mellitus. *N. Engl. J. Med.* **342**(19):1392-1398.

Cheney G. 1950. Anti-peptic ulcer dietary factor. *Journal of the American Dietetic Association* **26**:668-672.

Chernomorsky S. and Segelman A. 1988. Biological activities of chlorophyll derivatives. *New Jersey Medicine* **85**:669-673.

Choi H.K., Gao X. and Curhan G. 2009. Vitamin C Intake and the Risk of Gout in Men. *Archives of Internal Medicine* **169**(5):502–507.

Clayton E.T. 1962. How to live longer. *Ebony* **17**(12):110-117.

Colio L. and Babb V. 1948. Study of stimulatory growth

factor. *Journal of Biological Chemistry* **174**:405-409.

Collings G. 1945. Chlorophyll and adrenal cortical extract in the local treatment of burns. *American Journal of Surgery* **70**:58-63.

Combs G.F. 2008. *The Vitamins: Fundamental Aspects in Nutrition and Health*. Elsevier, San Diego.

Council on Food and Nutrition 1962. The regulation of dietary fat. *Journal of the American Medical Association* **181**(5):411-429.

Corbett J.V. 1995. Accidental poisoning with iron supplements. *MCN Am. J. Matern Child Nur.* **20**(4):234.

Cumler W.V. *Physical Fitness Program for Men.* Y.M.C.A. Central Branch, Cleveland, Ohio.

Dallman P.R. 1986. Biochemical basis for the manifestations of iron deficiency. *Annual Rev. Nutr.* **6:**13-40.

Dahm C.C., Keogh R.H., Spencer E.A., Greenwood D.C., Key T.J., Fentiman I.S., Shipley M.J., Brunner E.J., Cade J.E., Burley V.J. Mishra G., Stephen A.M., Kuh D., White I.R., Luben R., Lentjes M.A., Khaw K.T. and Rodwell Bingham S.A. 2010. Dietary fiber and colorectal cancer risk: a nested case-control study using food diaries. *J. Natl. Cancer Inst.* **102**(9):614-626.

de Vogel J., Jonker-Termont D.S.M.L., Katan M.B. and van der Meer R. 2005. Natural Chlorophyll but Not Chlorophyllin Prevents Heme-Induced Cytotoxic and Hyperproliferative Effects in Rat Colon. *J. Nutr.* (The American Society for Nutritional Sciences) **135**(8):1995–2000.

de Vogel J., Jonker-Termont D.S.M.L., van Lieshout E.M., Katan M.B. and van der Meer R. 2005. Green vegetables, red meat and colon cancer: chlorophyll prevents the cytotoxic and hyperproliferative effects of haem in rat colon. *Carcinogenesis* **26**:387-393.

Do M.H., Lee S.S., Jung P.J. and Lee M.H. 2007. Intake of fruits, vegetables, and soy foods in relation to breast cancer risk in Korean women: a case-control study. *Nutr. Cancer.* **57**(1):20-27.

Dublin L.I. and Marks H.H. 1958. *Mortality among Insured Overweights in Recent Years.* In: Ungerleider H.E. and Gubner R. (Eds.) *Life Insurance Medicine* Springfield, III: Charles C. Thomas, pp. 436-462.

Duffus C.M. and Duffus J.H. 1984. *Carbohydrate Metabolism in Plants.* Longman. London and New

York.

Dunne L.J. 2002. *Nutrition Almanac* (5th Ed.). McGraw-Hill, New York.

Eastwood M. 1987. Dietary fiber and the risk of cancer. *Nutrition Reviews* **45**:193-197.

Eckstein R.W. 1957. Effect of exercise and coronary artery narrowing on coronary collateral circulation. *Circ. Res.* **5**(3): 230-235.

Fahey J.W., Stephenson K.K., Dinkova-Kostova A.T., Egner P.A., Kensler T.W. and Talalay P. 2005. Chlorophyll, chlorophyllin and related tetrapyrroles are significant inducers of mammalian phase 2 cytoprotective genes. *Carcinogenesis* **26**(7):1247–1255.

Farmer B., Larson B.T., Fulgoni V.L. 3rd, Rainville A.J. and Liepa G.U. 2011. A vegetarian dietary pattern as a nutrient-dense approach to weight management: an analysis of the national health and nutrition examination survey 1999-2004. *J. Am. Diet Assoc.* **11**(6):819-827.

Ferruzzi M.G. and Blakesleeb J. 2007. Digestion, absorption, and cancer preventative activity of dietary chlorophyll derivatives. *Nutrition Research* **27**(1): 1–12.

Ferruzzi M.G., Böhm V., Courtney P. and Schwartz S.J. 2002. Antioxidant and antimutagenic activity of dietary chlorophyll derivatives determined by radical scavenging and bacterial reverse mutagenesis assays. *J. Food Sci.* **67**:2589–2595.

Fleuret A. 1979. The role of wild foliage plants in the diet; a case study from Lushoto, Tanzania. *Ecology of Food and Nutrition* **8**:87-93.

Freeman J.M., Kossf E.H. and Hartman A.L. 2007. The Ketogenic Diet: One Decade Later. *Pediatrics* **119**(3):535-543.

Freud S. 1933. *New Introductory Lectures on Psychoanalysis.* Penguin Freud Library 2, pp. 105-106.

Fukuwatari T. and Shibata K. 2008. Urinary water-soluble vitamins and their metabolite contents as nutritional markers for evaluating vitamin intakes in young Japanese women. *J. Nutr. Sci. Vitaminol.* **54**(3):223–229.

Gershwin M., Beach R. and Hurley L. 1985. *Nutrition and Immunity.* Academic Press. Orlando.

Gilbody S., Lewis S., Lightfoot T. 2007. Methylenetetrahydrofolate reductase (MTHFR) genetic polymorphisms and psychiatric disorders: a HuGE review. *American Journal of Epidemiology* **165**(1):1–13.

Goldberg G. (Ed.) 2003. *Plants: Diet and Health*. British Nutrition Society. Blackwell Science, Oxford, UK.

Graham W., Kohler G. and Schnabel C. 1940. *Grass as a Food: Vitamin Content*. Paper presented April 10, 1940, at the 99th meeting of The American Chemical Society.

Griffin J.P. (Ed.). 2009 *The Textbook of Pharmaceutical Medicine* (6th Ed.). Wiley-Blackwell, New Jersey.

Grisham C.M. and Reginald H.G. 1999. *Biochemistry*. Saunders College Pub., Philadelphia, pp. 426–427.

Gruskin B. 1940. Chlorophyll — its therapeutic place in acute and suppurative disease. *American Journal of Surgery* **49**:49-55.

Guthrie H.A. 1983. *Introductory Nutrition* (5th Ed.). The C.V. Mosby Co., St. Louis, 675pp.

Haas J.D. and Brownlie T. 4th 2001. Iron deficiency and reduced work capacity: a critical review of the research to determine a causal relationship. *J Nutr.* **131**(2S-2):676S-6905.

Hagiwara Y. 1985. *Green Barley Essence, The Ideal Fast Food*. Keats Publishing, New Canaan, Connecticut.

Hamilton E., Whitney E. and Sizer F. 1988. *Nutrition: Concepts and Controversies* (4th Ed.). West Publishing Co. St. Paul, Minn.

Hammel-Dupont C. and Bessman S. 1970. The stimulation of hemoglobin synthesis by porphyrins. *Biochemical Medicine* **4**:55-60.

Hiroko S. 2001. History and characteristics of Okinawan longevity food. *Asia Pacific J. Clin. Nutr.* **10**(2):159–164.

Hou J.K., Abraham B. and El-Serag H. 2011. Dietary intake and risk of developing inflammatory bowel disease: a systematic review of the literature. *Am. J. Gastroenterol.* **106**(4):563-573.

Howell E. 1980. *Food Enzymes for Health and Longevity*. Omangod Press, Woodstock Valley, CT.

Hughes J. and Latner A. 1936. Chlorophyll and haemoglobin regeneration after haemorrhage. *Journal of Physiology* **86**:388-395.

Institute of Medicine 2005. *Dietary Reference Intakes for*

Energy, Carbohydrate, Fiber, Fat, Fatty Acids, Cholesterol, Protein, and Amino Acids. National Academies Press Washington DC.

Institute of Medicine 2010. *Dietary Reference Intakes for Calcium and Vitamin* D. Committee to Review Dietary Reference Intakes for Vitamin D and Calcium. Food and Nutrition Board. National Academy Press, Washington, DC.

Kephart J.C. 1955. Chlorophyll derivatives - chemistry, commercial preparations and uses. *Econ. Bot.* **9**:3–38.

Kimm S., Tschai B. and Park S. 1982. Antimutagenic activity of chlorophyll to direct and indirect-acting mutagens and its contents in the vegetables. *Korean Journal of Biochemistry* **14**:1-7.

Kochanek K.D., Xu J.Q., Murphy S.L., Miniño A.M. and Kung H.C. 2011. Deaths: Preliminary Data for 2009. National Center for Health Statistics. *National Vital Statistics Reports* **59**(4):68 pp.

Kohler G., Elvehjem C. and Hart E. 1936. Growth stimulating properties of grass juice. *Science* May 8, 445.

Kohler G. 1953. The unidentified vitamins of grass and

alfalfa. *Feedstuffs*, August 8, 1953.

Koo L. 1988. Dietary habits and lung cancer risk among Chinese females in Hong Kong who never smoked. *Nutrition and Cancer* **11**:155-172.

Kubota K., Matsuoka Y. and Seki, H. 1983. Isolation of potent anti-inflammatory protein from barley leaves. *Japanese Journal of Inflammation* **3**(4).

Kubota K. and Sunagane N. 1984. *Studies on the effects of green barley juice on the endurance and motor activity in mice.* Paper presented at The 104th Annual Congress of The Pharmaceutical Society of Japan in Sendai City, Japan.

La Vecchia C., Negri E., Decarli A., Davanzo B., and Franceschi S. 1987. A case-control study of diet and gastric cancer in Northern Italy. *International Journal of Cancer* **40**(4):484-489.

Lai C. 1978. Chlorophyll: The active factor in wheat sprout extract inhibiting the metabolic activation of carcinogens in vitro. *Nutritional Cancer* **1**:19-21.

Lai C., Butler M. and Matney T. 1980. Antimutagenic activities of common vegetables and their chlorophyll content. *Mutation Research* **77**:245-250.

Lakhanpal R., Davis J., Typpo J. and Briggs G. 1966. Evidence for an unidentified growth factor from alfalfa and other plant sources for young guinea pigs. *Journal of Nutrition* **89**:341-346.

Lam T.Y., Seto S.W., Au A.L., Poon C.C., Li R.W., Lam H.Y., Lau W.S., Chan S.W. *et al*. 2009. Folic acid supplementation modifies beta-adrenoceptor-mediated in vitro lipolysis of obese/diabetic (+db/+db) mice. *Experimental Biology and Medicine (Maywood, N.J.)* **234**(9):1047–1055.

Leklem J.E. 1999. Vitamin B6. In: *Modern Nutrition in Health and Disease*. (9th Ed.). Shils M.E., Olson J.A., Shike M. and Ross A.C. (Ed.). Williams and Wilkins, Baltimore, pp. 413-421.

Li Y. and Schellhorn H.E. 2007. New developments and novel therapeutic perspectives for vitamin C. *J. Nutr.* **137**:2171-2184.

Lieberman S. and Bruning N. 1990. *The Real Vitamin & Mineral Book*. Avery Group, New York.

Link L.B. and Potter J.D. 2004. Raw versus Cooked Vegetables and Cancer Risk. *Cancer Epidemiol. Biomarkers & Prevention* **13**(9):1422-35.

Locniskar M. 1988. Nutrition and Health Symposium: The University of Texas at Austin, April 1988, Summary Report. *Nutrition Today.* **Sept/Oct**:31-37.

Lonn E., Yusuf S., Arnold M.J., Sheridan P., Pogue J., Micks M., McQueen M.J., Probstfield J. *et al.* 2006. Homocysteine Lowering with Folic Acid and B Vitamins in Vascular Disease. *New England Journal of Medecine* **354**(15):1567–1577.

Marawaha R.K., Bansal D., Kaur S. and Trehan A. 2004. Wheatgrass Juice Reduces Transfusion Requirement in Patients with Thalassemia Major: A Pilot Study. *Indian Pediatric* **41**(7):716-720.

McBride J. 1999. Can foods forestall aging? *Agricultural Research* **47**(2):15-17.

McDougall J.A. 1985. *McDougall's Medicine: A Challenging Second Opinion.* New Century Publishers, Inc., New Jersey.

McEligot A.J., Largent J., Ziogas A., Peel D. and Anton-Culver H. 2006. Dietary fat, fiber, vegetable, and micronutrients are associated with overall survival in postmenopausal women diagnosed with breast cancer. *Nutr. Cancer* **55**(2):132-140.

Muto T. 1977. Therapeutic experiment of Bakuryokuso (Young Green Barley Juice) for the treatment of skin diseases in Man. *New Drugs and Clinical Application* **26**(5).

Nenonen M.T., Helve T.A., Rauma A.L. and Hänninen O.O. 1998. Uncooked, lactobacilli-rich, vegan food and rheumatoid arthritis. *Br. J. Rheumatol.* **37**(3):274-281.

Nesse R.M. and Williams G.C. 1996. *Why We Get Sick: New Science of Darwinian Medicine.* Times Books, New York.

Offenkrantz W. 1950. Water-soluble chlorophyll in the treatment of peptic ulcers of long duration. *Review of Gastroenterology* **17**:359-367.

Office of Dietary Supplements. Acc. 2011. *Dietary Supplements Fact Sheets.* United States Department of Health and Human Services, National Institutes of Health. http://ods.od.nih.gov/factsheets/list-all/ Accessed June 20, 2011.

Ohno Y., Yoshida O., Oishi K., Okada K., Yamabe H. and Schroeder F. 1988. Dietary beta-carotene and cancer of the prostate: a case-control study in Kyoto. *Cancer Research* **48**(5):1331-1336.

Olmedo J.M., Yiannias J.A., Windgassen E.B. and Gornet M.K. 2006. Scurvy: a disease almost forgotten. *Int. J. Dermatol.* **45**(8):909–913.

Ong T., Whong W., Stewart J. and Brockman H. 1986. Chlorophyllin: a potent antimutagen against environmental and dietary complex mixtures. *Mutation Research* **173**:111-15.

Otten J.J., Hellwig J.P. and Meyers L.D. (Eds.) 2006. *Diettary Reference Intakes: The Essential Guide to Nutrient Requirements.* Institute of Medicine of the National Academies. The National Academic Press, Washington DC.

Patek A. 1936. Chlorophyll and regeneration of the blood. *Archives of Internal Medicine* **57**:73-84.

Pirie N. 1969. The present position of research on the use of leaf protein as a human food. *Plant Foods and Human Nutrition* **1**:237-246.

Prior R.L., Hoang H., Gu L,. Wo X., Bacchocca M., Howard L., Hampsch-Woodill M., Huang D., Ou B. and Jacob R. 2003. Assays for hydrophilic and lipophylic antioxidant capacity (oxygen radical absorbance capacity (ORAC$_{FL}$)) of plasma and other biological and food samples. *J. Agric. Food Chem.*

51:3273-3279.

Price W. 2008. *Nutrition and Physical Degeneration*. Price-Pottenger Nutrition Foundation® (PPNF™), 527pp.

Potter J.D. 1999. Colorectal cancer: molecules and populations. *J. Natl. Cancer Inst.* **91**:916-932.

Raab W. 1961. Preventive medical mass reconditioning abroad – why not in U.S.A.? *Annals of Internal Medicine* **54**:1191-1208.

Raj A. and Katz M. 1985. Beta-carotene as an inhibitor of benzo(a)pyrene and mitomycin C induced chromosomal breaks in the bone marrow of mice. *Canadian Journal of Genetics and Cytology* **27**:598-602.

Refsum H., Ueland P.M., Nygard O. and Vollset S.E. 1998. Homocysteine and cardiovascular disease. *Annual Review of Medicine* **49**(1):31–62.

Rhoads J. 1939. The relation of vitamin K to the hemorrhagic tendency in obstructive jaundice with a report on cerophyll as a source of vitamin K. *Surgery* **5**:794-808.

Robinson A. 1979. Diet and Cancer. In: *Barron's Mailbag. Barron's*. September 3, 1993, p. 7.

Rosell M.S., Lloyd-Wright Z., Appleby P.N., Sanders T.A., Allen N.E. and Key T.J. 2005. Long-chain n-3 polyunsaturated fatty acids in plasma. *Am. J. Clin. Nutr.* **82**(2):327-334.

Rothemund P., McNary R. and Inman O. 1934. Occurrence of decomposition products of chlorophyll.II. Decomposition products of chlorophyll in the stomach walls of herbivorous animals. *Journal of the American Chemical Society* **56**:2400-2403.

Rothschild B. 2000. *The Body Remembers: The psychophysiology of Trauma and Trauma Treatment.* W.W. Norton & Company Inc., New York.

Sack P. and Barnard R. 1955. Studies on the hemagglutinating and inflammation properties of exudate from nonhealing wounds and their inhibition by chlorophyll derivatives. *New York State Journal of Medicine.* **15**: 2952-2956.

Sapolsky R.M. 2004. *Why Zebras Don't Get Ulcers* (3rd Ed.). Owl Books, New York.

Schnabel C. 1935. *The biologic value of high protein cereal grasses.* Paper presented to the Biologic Section of the American Chemical Society in New York, April 22, 1935.

Scott E. and Delor C. 1933. Nutritional anemia. *Ohio State Medical Journal* **29**:165-169.

Scott M. 1986. *Nutrition of Humans and Selected Animal Species*. John Wiley and Sons, New York.

Segerstrom S.C. and Miller G.E. 2004. Psychological stress and the immune system: a meta-analytical study of 30-years of inquiry. *Psichol. Bull* **130**(4):601-630.

Seibold R.L. (Ed.) 2003. *Cereal Grass. What's In It For You!* PINES International, Inc., Lawrence, Kansas, USA. http://wheatgrass.com/t-cgbook.aspx Accessed May 11, 2011.

Sho H. 2001. History and Characteristics of Okinawan Longevity Food. *Asia Pacific Journal of Clinical Nutrition.* **10**:159-164.

Singh K., Pannu M.S., Singh P. and Singh J. 2010. Effect of wheat grass tablets on the frequency of blood transfusions in Thalassemia Major. *Indian J. Pediatr.* **77**(1):90-91.

Smith A.L. 1997. *Oxford dictionary of biochemistry and molecular biology*. Oxford University Press, Oxford, p. 508.

Smith L. 1944. Chlorophyll: an experimental study of its water-soluble derivatives. Remarks on the history, chemistry, toxicity and anti-bacterial properties of water soluble chlorophyll as therapeutic agents. *American Journal of the Medical Sciences* **207**:647-654.

Smith L. 1955. The present status of topical chlorophyll therapy. *The NY State Journal of Medicine* **15**: 2041-2049.

Spector H. and Calloway D. 1959. Reduction of x-radiation mortality by cabbage and broccoli. *Proceedings of the Society for Experimental Biology and Medicine* **100**:405-407.

Stahl W., Heinrich U., Jungmann H. *et al.* 1998. Increased Dermal Carotenoid Levels Assessed by Noninvasive Reflection Spectrophotometry Correlate with Serum Levels in Women Ingesting Betatene. *Journal of Nutrition* **128**(5):903–907.

Steinmetz K.A. and Potter J.D. 1996. Vegetables, fruit and cancer prevention: a review. *J. Am. Diet. Assoc.* **96**:1027–1039.

Subar A., Block G. and James L. 1989. Folate intake and food sources in the U.S. population. *American Journal of Clinical Nutrition* **50**:508-516.

Thomas K.B. 1987. General Practice consultations: is there any point in being positive? *British Medical Journal* **294**: 1200-1202.

USDA/ARS (U.S. Department of Agriculture, Agricultural Research Service) 2010. *Oxygen Radical Absorbance Capacity (ORAC) of Selected Foods*, Release 2. Nutrient Data Laboratory. Home Page: http://www.ars.usda.gov/nutrientdata/orac Accessed on July 1, 2011.

USDA/HHS (U.S.Department of Agriculture and U.S. Department of Health and Human Services) 2010. *Dietary Guidelines for Americans 2010* (7th Ed.). U.S. Government Printing Office, Washington DC, 95pp.

Valtin H. 2002. "Drink at least eight glasses of water a day." Really? Is there Scientific Evidence for "8X8"? *American Journal of Physiology* **283**:993-1004.

Verreault R., Chu J., Mandelson M. and Shy K. 1989. A case-control study of diet and invasive cervical cancer. *International Journal of Cancer* **43**(6):1050-1054.

Voet D. and Voet J.G. 2004. *Biochemistry* Vol 1 (3rd Ed.). Hoboken, Wiley, N.J.

Walford R. and Walford L. 2005. *The Caloric Limitation Principle, Review: The Anti-Aging Plan: The Nutrient-Rich, Low-Calorie Way of Eating for a Longer Life - The Only Diet Scientifically Proven to Extend Your Healthy Years*. Da Capo Press, Cambridge, Mass., pp. 26–27.

WHO – World Health Organization. Acc. 2011. Global Stategy on Diet, Physical Activity and Health. http://www.who.int/dietphysicalactivity/diet/en/index.html Accessed on 10-06-2011.

Wigmore A. 1985. *The Wheatgrass Book*. D. Puglisi (Ed.). AVERY, Penguin Putman Inc., 126pp.

Willcox B.J., Willcox D.C. and Suzuki M. 2005. *The Okinawa Diet Plan: Get Leaner, Live Longer, and Never Feel Hungry* . Three Rivers Press, New York.

Willcox B.J., Willcox D.C., Todoriki H., Fujiyoshi A., Yano K., He Q., Curb J.D. and Suzuki M. 2007. Caloric restriction, the traditional Okinawan diet, and healthy aging: the diet of the world's longest-lived people and its potential impact on morbidity and life span. *Annals of the New York Academy of Sciences* **1114**:434–455.

Woolley D. and Krampitz L. 1943. Production of a scurvy-like condition by feeding of a compound structurally related to ascorbic acid. *Journal of*

Experimental Medicine **78**:333.

Young R.W. and Beregi J.S. 1980. Use of chlorophyll in the care of geriatric patients. *Journal of the American Geriatric Society* **28**(1):46-47.

Yu Y.M., Chang W.C., Chang C.T., Hsieh C.L. and Tsai C.E. 2002. Effects of young barley leaf extract and antioxidative vitamins on LDL oxidation and free radical scavenging activities in type 2 diabetes. *Diabetes & Metabolism* **28**(2):107-714.

Yu Y.M., Wu C.H., Tseng Y.H., Tsai C.E. and Chang W.C. 2002. Antioxidative and hypolipidemic effects of barley leaf essence in a rabbit model of atherosclerosis. *Japanese Journal of Pharmacology* **89**(2): 142-148.

Zhang C.X., Ho S.C., Chen Y.M., Fu J.H., Cheng S.Z. and Lin F.Y. 2009. Greater vegetable and fruit intake is associated with a lower risk of breast cancer among Chinese women. *Int. J. Cancer* **125**(1):181-188.

Ziegler R., Mason T., Stemhagen A., Hoover R., Schoenberg J., Gridley G., Virgo P. and Fraumeni J. 1986. Carotenoid intake, vegetables, and the risk of lung cancer among white men in New Jersey. *American Journal of Epidemiology* **123**:1080-1093.

Zittoun J. 1993. Anemias due to disorder of folate, vitamin B12 and transcobalamin metabolism. *Rev. Prat.* **43**:1358-1363.

www.ingramcontent.com/pod-product-compliance
Lightning Source LLC
Chambersburg PA
CBHW060246290526
45789CB00001B/211